Ooh Matron!

By

Sarah Jane Butfield

Copyright

©2015 Sarah Jane Butfield

©2015 Clair Victoria Butfield – Chapter twelve Student nurse training now.

Cover design: Amygdala design

Editor: Martin Papworth

First paperback edition: September 2015.

ISBN-13: 978-1515398233

ISBN-10: 1515398234

The moral right of the author has been asserted. All rights reserved. No part of this book may be reproduced, stored in a retrieval system or transmitted in any form or by any means, electronic, mechanical, photocopying, or otherwise without the written permission of the author and publisher.

The people and events portrayed in this book are as remembered, perceived and/or experienced by Sarah Jane Butfield. However, some of the names and locations have been changed for privacy and legal reasons. The author takes no responsibility for the accuracy of events and dialogue retold to her by third parties, close friends or family.

The photographs included in this book include some recovered scanned copies, as we lost most of our originals in the Australian floods, hence the production quality may be impaired. Other photographs have been obtained and used with the permission of family and friends, including Samantha Parker and Richard Klein.

For links to all of Sarah Jane's books and to join her private mailing list for subscriber first access to sneak previews and behind the scenes photographs visit Sarah Jane's author website

Contents

Copyright

Dedication

Acknowledgements

Introduction

Chapter one:
What do you want to be when you grow up?

Chapter two:
Student Nurse McDonald

Chapter three:
Banana Banshee Happy Hour

Chapter four:
Mind your backs!

Chapter five:
Slip, slop, slap summer fun

Chapter six:
Wacky races and sad faces

Chapter seven:
Do I really want to be a nurse?

Chapter eight:
Highs and lows of womanhood revealed

Chapter nine:
Mind Matters

Chapter ten:

Theatrical high jinks and honey traps

Chapter eleven:

By Royal appointment

Chapter twelve:

Student nurse training now

Chapter thirteen:

Accident and Emergency beckons

Chapter fourteen:

The Anatomy of becoming a qualified nurse

Chapter fifteen:

Enter Staff Nurse Parker

Medical Terms Glossary

Step back in time

About the author

Travel Memoirs by Sarah Jane Butfield

Other books by Sarah Jane Butfield

Sneak preview: Bedpans to Boardrooms!

Dedication

This book is dedicated to the many people who inspired and nurtured me and my career during my formative years as a nurse. However, in addition, I would like to dedicate it to student nurses and nursing assistants for their contribution to healthcare, in its many forms, around the world. The nursing profession is not an island and it takes a team effort to provide consistently high standards of care. To nurse educators and ward based mentors in all specialties who play such a vital part in laying the foundations for high quality nursing care provision for our future generations. And last but by no means least to the ancillary staff who support all grades of staff, not just by fulfilling their roles to the highest standard, but by being the ones to go the extra mile for you. For example, from my experiences they will be the ones to bring you a cup of coffee when you have already worked eight hours with no official break and still have at least four hours to go. Or those who come to your aid when a patient gets violent or abusive towards you while help is summoned.

Thank you to everyone, you are all appreciated.

Over the years a couple of nursing based quotes have become memorable for me and I would like to share those here in case anyone else can relate to them:

'Sometimes I inspire my patients; more often they inspire me.' Unknown author.

'They may forget your name, but they will never forget how you made them feel.' - Maya Angelou.

'Nurses may not be angels, but they are the next best thing.' Anonymous.

Acknowledgements

Firstly I would like to say a big thank you to my editor Martin Papworth. An honest, gracious and hardworking gentleman who has enhanced my work and reputation as an author. Secondly to Clair Victoria Butfield, my step-daughter and newly qualified paediatric staff nurse who kindly contributed to this book to provide a comparison between student nurse training in Essex 1983-1986 versus 2012-2015.

I would also like to acknowledge and thank the following people and groups for helping me on my writing journey to date and providing the support and encouragement I needed to expand my memoir writing into a new direction with this new nursing and medical memoir series. Just knowing that your peers have faith in your writing ability can carry an author a very long way.

My social media friends and colleagues in the Rukia Publishing social media tweet team including the leaders, Nigel Butfield, Samantha Parker & Shontae Brewster.
http://www.rukiapublishing.com/

'We Love Memoirs' Facebook Group and especially Julie Haigh for her input towards the cover design for this book and her relentless endeavours to support the WLM authors. Julie also provides a tremendous source of help and guidance to myself and many of the WLM authors on Goodreads which is greatly appreciated.
https://www.facebook.com/groups/welovememoirs/

'Tom Winton Authors Helping Authors' Facebook Group especially Tom Winton and Mark Williams.
https://www.facebook.com/groups/495847367109155/

ASMSG - Author Social Media Support Group, its tweet teams and the inspirational Christoph Fischer.
https://www.facebook.com/groups/389343847782037/

Ooh Matron!

Introduction

'Ooh Matron!' is the first book in The Nomadic Nurse Series which serves as a biographical compilation of stories, anecdotes and reflections from a varied nursing career in health care establishments across the UK and in various parts of Australia.

Each book in this series will represent a new chapter or episode in my nursing career, which I hope will not only be entertaining, but may also inspire readers to explore all opportunities, however obscure they may at first appear.

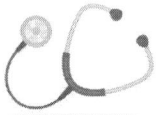

Sarah Jane has no career aspirations, all she wants is to leave school, work as a cashier at Woolworths and get married. Then everything changes and she finds herself wearing a fluorescent pink uniform and studying to get into Nursing School. What inspired this surprising change of direction? What happens when she leaves home to live in a garrison town with a housemate who is a party animal? The big question being, is she really cut out to be a nurse?

Let's start at the beginning with Sarah Jane as a sixteen-year-old country girl, a bit old-fashioned but who has a mischievous sense of humour who suddenly decides she wants to be a nurse!

Beta reader review

"This funny, yet poignant nursing memoir has Sarah Jane's trademark honest writing style which shines through in every story she tells. From starting her student nurse training in Essex to coping with patients in happy, sad and heart-breaking situations. It gives you a young woman's view into the realities of entering the world of nursing in the 1980's. A highly entertaining and informative memoir which was able to take me from laughing out loud to having welled tears of empathy." S. Brewster.

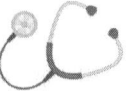

Why is it called 'Ooh Matron' and what does that bring to mind for you? Readers of a certain age will probably remember the naughty seaside postcard style humour of the 'Carry On' films series in the 1960s, 70s and 80s. The films starred some of the great comedy actors of all time such as Kenneth Williams, Barbara Windsor, Sid James, Jim Dale, Frankie Howerd and Hattie Jacques, to name but a few. I grew up exposed to these films as my mum was a huge fan. She had a wonderful, infectious, slightly naughty laugh, so this type of humour entertained her. My mum's love and fondness for Hattie Jacques originated from these humble beginnings. She watched all the films that Hattie appeared in many times over, her favourites being '*Carry On Matron*' and '*Carry On Doctor*'.

There was a physical resemblance between my mum and Hattie Jacques, but in hindsight and with a tinge of sadness I realise now that they were also similar in their personalities and the personal struggles they faced with relationships, weight gain and loss.

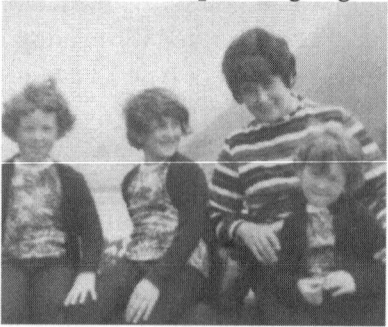

My Mum, me and two of my sisters
From left to right Susie, me, mum and Sally

Ooh Matron!

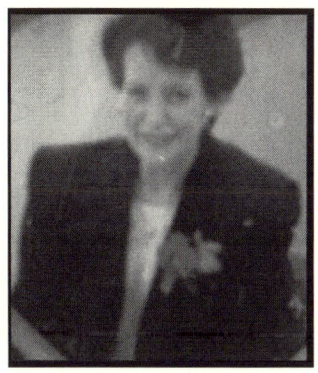

Our mum in 1990

One of the proudest moments of my life was the day I told my mum I had passed my final examinations and was at last a qualified nurse, even though she didn't see why I needed a career as I had 'a nice man to take care of me'. Nevertheless, I knew that she was proud of me and if she were alive today and had witnessed the twists and turns of my twenty-eight year nursing career I think she would have become one of those annoying neighbours always going on about their super talented offspring. Everything that I have achieved over the years is due in part to the sacrifices she made both on both a physical and psychological level during my childhood. I hope she knows that those sacrifices were worth it and that as a result I have managed to provide for my children over the years with the security of a valuable nursing qualification behind me.

So let's start at the beginning with my innocent days of becoming and living the student nurse life in Colchester, Essex. Find out how and why a sixteen-year-old country girl, who was a bit old-fashioned, but had a mischievous sense of humour, suddenly decided she wanted to be a nurse!

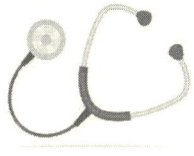

Chapter one:
What do you want to be when you grow up?

In 1981, as I neared completion of my high school years in Debenham, Suffolk, I had no thoughts about a career of any description. I knew that I would need to find a job straight away because we would need the money and I wanted my mum to work less. However, I had no thoughts of finding a career, considering what direction it might take and where that decision would lead me in the future. As a young country girl growing up with typically traditional, some would say, old-fashioned family values instilled by my mum, I always imagined leaving school and working as a cashier in Woolworths or one of the another department stores in the nearby town of Ipswich. This would be followed eventually by getting married and having a family of my own to care for. There was never any mention or discussion about me pursuing a career of any description and, with no career motivated role models to inspire that train of thought, I had no deep rooted ambitions or objectives, because that wasn't how my life was destined to be.

I came from a family where my mum, a single parent, not by preference but as a result of a poor choice in men, worked three jobs in the days of little or no social security support. She worked as a cleaner, regularly undertook a variety of fruit and vegetable picking jobs, turkey plucking at the local farm before Christmas and she also worked as home carer. She did all of this to ensure that myself and my three sisters always had everything that we needed. We did not have an extended family network to rely on apart from my Nan, who lived in the next village, however, she had limited mobility, using two walking sticks due to chronic leg ulcers, but she loved having me there to watch the wrestling on television with her on Saturday afternoon.

Unless I was oblivious to it, there was little talk of careers at school until towards the end of the final year and it was after one of the first sessions with the careers adviser that I thought, 'Hey perhaps there is more on offer than a shop job.' At one of the sessions we had a talk from a tutor from the Suffolk College who handed out the prospectus for the coming year. I turned the pages not even sure what I was looking for. True to my old-fashioned approach to life, thinking of jobs suitable for women, I headed straight for the secretarial office skills section. This was before I remembered the words of my office studies teacher Mrs Sibley, "You might be better suited to filing and indexing than typing, so let's not worry about the typing speed and accuracy test."

Several of my friends were opting for hairdressing courses, but I had always been such a 'Tom-Boy' with little interest in anything of that nature and always happiest in my dungarees sporting my usual unkempt hair style or a ponytail.

One definition of a 'Tom boy' is:
"A girl who behaves in a way that is perceived to be stereotypically boyish or masculine and/or a girl who acts or dresses in a boyish way, liking rough outdoor activities."
Quote http://www.thefreedictionary.com/tomboy

This definitely applied to me, a born and bred country girl. As I turned the page I saw a photograph of an elderly man being helped to put his socks on, in what looked like his own home, by a pre-nursing student wearing an extremely bright, almost fluorescent pink uniform dress. Something stirred in my brain. No, not the thought of the pink dress. At once this image made me think of my Nan and her leg ulcers and how the district nurse visited each week, sometimes with a helper, to redress them. I also thought about our elderly neighbour Mr Forsyth whom I visited a couple of times a week to apply or check on his corn plasters. He couldn't reach to do it himself due to his arthritic knees and hips, or his war wounds as he called them. My mum had done some home carer work so perhaps I could do something similar after completing this course. I liked old people, they were interesting and always had great stories to tell.

This accidental and humble beginning is where it all began, and so my nursing journey started.

Sarah Jane Butfield

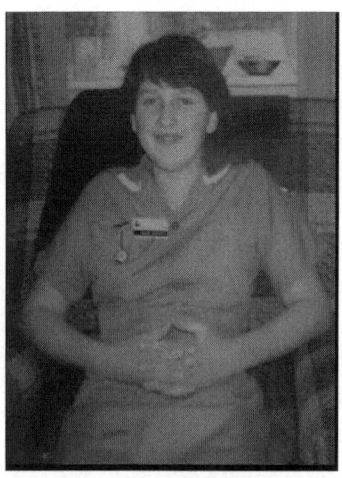

Don't I look the part in my pink pre-nursing student uniform, fob watch and identity badge?

In September 1981 I started the pre-nursing course at Suffolk College in Ipswich. The purpose of the course was to prepare students for making an application to any UK nursing training establishment to complete either their State Enrolled Nurse (SEN) or State Registered Nurse (SRN) training, I wasn't entirely sure I would do either of those, but I focused on completing the course and achieving the entry qualifications anyway. The course that I was accepted onto aimed to incorporate the educational elements to ensure that all students achieved the minimum of five O levels including Mathematics and English language at Grade C or above, which was the minimum entry qualification for an SRN training place, although some training hospitals required more and higher qualifications especially if places were heavily oversubscribed. This was often the case at the prestigious London hospitals and what today would be called 'Centres of Excellence'.

O level was the shortened term for ordinary level, as opposed to A level which was advanced level, examinations in a variety of subjects. Today's equivalent qualifications are known as GSCE's, an abbreviation for General Certificate of Secondary Education.

At the end of my schooling, my examination tally was a meagre one O level Grade B in English Language. I needed another four, so I signed up to study Mathematics, General Science, Biology, Human

Biology and Sociology as my core subjects. We took part in a half day per week pre nursing placement at the local hospital wards, units and clinics to enable us to observe and eventually participate in physical patient care activities. I enjoyed college life, mainly because it differed from school where I was not one of the popular girls and to be honest I dreaded going most days. Today we would probably label it bullying, but in those days it was just kids being unkind to each other or picking on the overweight girl in the class wearing the second-hand blazer. In college with no uniform to worry about and the ability to find your own friends either within your classmates or from other courses, the pressure lifted and the social elements kicked in. However, perhaps that wasn't a good thing. At the end of year one, when the examination results arrived, I was disappointed to have only passed my Mathematics and General Science exams with a Grade B in both which meant I still didn't have the entry qualifications.

I debated changing to the SEN course which at the time only need two or three passes, but at seventeen years old and still too young to start my nurse training anyway I thought I might as well give it another shot and do another full year. As a second year pre-nursing student I upgraded to completing a full day on placement each week. I really enjoyed this especially as I had some home-care and rehabilitation unit placements. I also decided that this was the year to put the work in and increase the odds of achieving the desired grades. Therefore, I studied for five O levels this year which included repeating Biology, Human Biology and Sociology and adding new subjects History of Nursing and Physics. In addition, I studied for Chemistry and English Literature at evening classes; surely I would pass two out of seven.

About six months before examination time I applied for nursing courses to Ipswich and Colchester, despite my classmates applying to hospitals around the UK. After an interview and entry test I was offered a place at the Colchester School of Nursing subject to achieving the required five O level passes. As it turned out I learned that if I apply myself I can achieve more than I ever imagined possible. I passed all seven O levels with grades A and B meaning I now had ten, double the required amount. This achievement won

Sarah Jane Butfield

me an Award of Merit which made my mum extremely proud. She kept a copy of the newspaper clipping and the acceptance ceremony photograph on her drinks cabinet until the day she died.

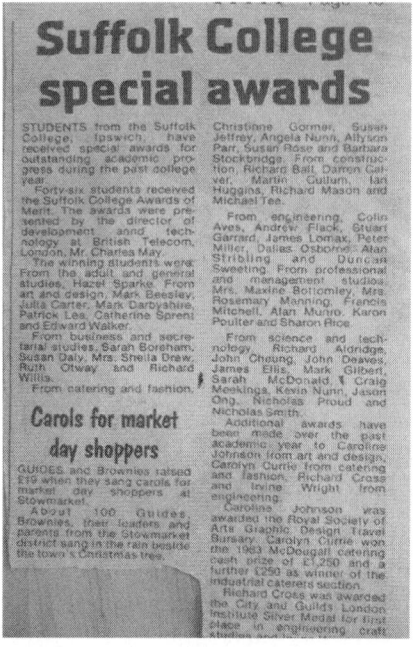

The list of award winners in the Evening Star Newspaper

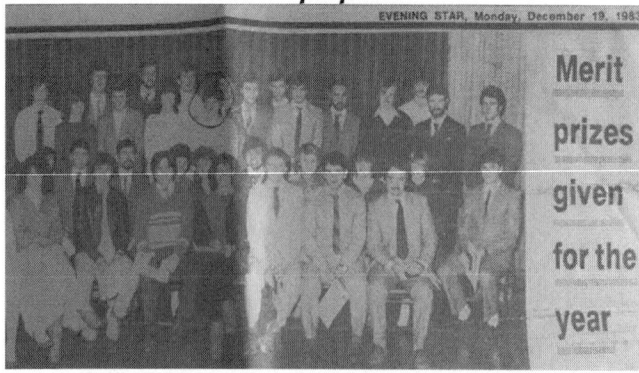

The group photograph after the awards ceremony

Ooh Matron!

The thought crossed my mind that I could consider a London hospital after all instead of staying local. This flash of ambition was short lived as I already had a long-term boyfriend who wasn't thrilled at the idea and made no secret of it. After formally accepting my place as a student nurse at the Colchester School of Nursing I received a start date for October 1983. I would now move on to the next stage of my nursing career which could begin in earnest.

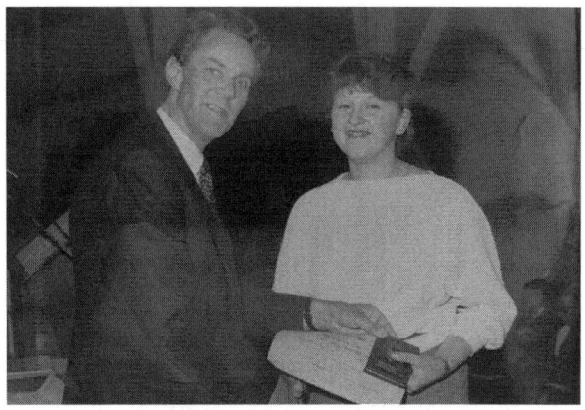

Accepting my award of Merit

The award

Chapter two:
Student Nurse McDonald

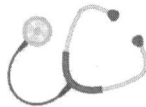

It was 10th October 1983, and after two years at college everything started to change. Until now the only jobs I could claim on my Curriculum Vitae or resumé included part time waitress, bar maid, summer holiday fruit picker and Christmas holiday turkey-plucker. These colourful job titles would soon be superseded by the status of student nurse at Colchester School of Nursing. The time had come to not only leave home, but to start three years of training to become a qualified general nurse. My new home would be in Colchester which, although situated only nineteen miles from Ipswich, in 1983 for an eighteen year old who didn't drive, proved impossible to get to for a variety of shift times and patterns spread over the seven days of the week.

Classified as a 'remote student' because I lived with my family in Ipswich, I qualified for hospital staff accommodation at a subsidised rate which would be deducted at source from my earnings. The pre-employment paperwork confirmed that I had been allocated a room in a shared hospital house situated in Mill Road to the rear of Severalls Hospital. The majority of the hospital provided the psychiatric services for both in and out patients with a small part allocated to general hospital care services, including surgery, medical and respiratory wards. The hospital grounds were also home to the Colchester School of Nursing classrooms and library. After the closure of Severalls Hospital in the late 1990s, the education unit, part of the North East Essex Health Authority, became affiliated to the Anglia Ruskin University in Chelmsford and nursing students achieved degree status upon qualification. With its long history in psychiatric care and experimentation originating from its asylum days, the hospital has many features

Ooh Matron!

and stories which I found really insightful. For any readers interested in the asylum history of the hospital, formerly known as the Second Essex County Asylum and Severalls Mental Hospital and the part it played in the 1950s psychiatric experiments including lobotomies, there is a supplementary chapter called, 'Step back in time' at the end of this book.

Use of the phrase 'nerve-wracking' to describe the day I left home and moved into the hospital accommodation probably sounds dramatic, but at eighteen years old a little drama is allowed. The emotional process of saying my goodbyes to my mum and my sisters turned out to be one of the hardest parts of this new adventure that I was starting out on. You would be forgiven for thinking that I was in the process of moving to the other side of the world given my age, immaturity and blatant emotional outbursts. The reality in fact was that I would be only thirty to forty minutes away by car which now sounds ridiculous. However, at the time, neither I, my mum, nor my sisters had a car so that analogy carried no weight on the way I viewed my situation. This next part however would be even more daunting, a step into the unknown, living alone away from home. I would not be moving into the comfort of a setting up home with my boyfriend or husband, which is how I always imagined the day I left home would be. No, this would be a whole new ball game. My boyfriend Keith collected me and my belongings from home in Ipswich and as we turned off the A12 and drove into Colchester the reality what was happening suddenly kicked in.

We drove to Severalls Hospital, as per the instructions in my starter pack, and picked up an envelope from the Porter's Office. The envelope contained a letter and a shiny silver coloured Yale door key with blue plastic tag labelled number SN/58MR. The hand written letter contained a crude pencil drawn map with a star marking the location of the property. The letter said that I had been allocated a room upstairs and that my room key would be hanging in the entrance hall at the property.

The hospital accommodation was a semi-detached house with three bedrooms, which would have made a lovely family home. I would discover that, instead, the three bedrooms and the room at the front downstairs, which would have been the lounge, had been made into individual bed-sits for students and newly qualified nurses. Not that I considered myself to be a nurse at that stage, I didn't even have a uniform! As I unlocked and opened the front door the first thing I noticed was that the entire length of the hallway was scattered with shoes of all shapes, sizes and type. High heeled fashion boots, shoes, slippers and even some wellington boots and most of them not in pairs or in any kind of order. I wondered how many people lived there or if a big group of people were visiting. Behind the door, slightly hindering it from opening fully a row of wall-mounted coat hooks visibly strained, with wall plugs slightly protruding out of the plasterboard wall, under the weight of nurse's capes, raincoats jumpers, anoraks and shopping bags.

    My boyfriend Keith stood in the hall near the front door looking a bit scared. He eventually followed me. The only room key hanging in the hall, as we let ourselves in, was labelled 'upstairs – Room 2'. The carpeted stairs were in dire need of a vacuum, as dust and fluff had accumulated in each corner of every stair tread. At the top of the stairs there were four doors. Three with numbers on and the other sporting an old-fashioned porcelain plaque with the word *'Bathroom'* and a painted yellow duck illustration. My room, number two was to my right as I reached the landing. I used the key from the entrance hall to open the lock and went inside. My first impression was that there must have been a mistake because the room did not look ready for a new arrival. The evidence suggested movement from room two to room four at the back of the house. This evidence came in the form of an incriminating trail of tissues and dusty fluff balls along the hallway landing area thus exposing the culprit. One of the other house mates had obviously taken the opportunity to move rooms when one had become free. According to the information pack three other student nurses lived here.

    Basic is the most accurate word I can use to describe my room. A single bed, a three drawer unit hand basin with a small oval mirror above it and a big window which faced the road covered by a yellow stained net curtain. The bed, unmade with no bedding in sight, and the carpet scattered with hole-punch waste paper circles, paperclips and hairgrips, formed a daunting image. It's no wonder

Ooh Matron!

they hadn't used the vacuum in there. I felt very lost and really wanted to cry, but I didn't want to upset Keith before he left, which was rather quickly, and this upset me a bit more. I sat on the unmade bed and cried when he left.

This sudden sense of being lonely, small and inadequate heightened when I heard what I presumed to be the other house mates arrive home within a few minutes of Keith leaving. I wondered if they had seen or spoken to him as he left the house. I don't know why, but I presumed they were in their rooms studying or sleeping when I arrived as the house was so quiet. Now congregating in the hall and kitchen by the sounds of their voices, they talked about questions in the Hospital Final's examination and what they planned to do that evening. I opened my door a little wider to try to listen harder and to work out how many voices I could hear. However, they obviously heard the door creak because they ran up the stairs like excited kids hearing an ice cream van in the street on a hot sunny day. Before I had chance to move or do anything there they were in front of me, all wearing their nurse uniforms and standing looking at me. I immediately also realised that my makeup and mascara, diluted by my tears, made it obvious that I had been crying because Josie, whose room was downstairs lunged forward and hugged me. As I would discover over the coming weeks, Josie was the extrovert, party animal of the house. She was tall, with dark, short cropped hair and large brown eyes.

"Don't cry sweetie, we don't bite," she said.

The other two girls were different in both physical appearance and their personalities. Tracy had long dark hair, which she had released from its hair band during my uncomfortably elongated hug from Josie. She said hello, introduced herself and pointed to her room, number 3, then left. Tracy was a classic biker chick, wore no makeup and had an extremely pale complexion. Karen, the third girl, had short spiky hair and piercing blue eyes, which for some reason made me feel uneasy. After a short introduction, she didn't hang around either. I later discovered she had moved out of my room to take the room that I had been allocated, number four. So that was that. With the introductions over, Josie helped me to find some bed linen and gave me a tour of the house while she chattered continuously about the local pubs, her recent dates in intimate detail and her plans for when she qualified in the next couple of months.

The tour of the shared kitchen became quite comical in hindsight, but at the time it shocked me as it was nothing like our kitchen at home or any that I had worked in. There was a combined fridge freezer tucked into an alcove near to the back door, with each of us supposedly allocated a shelf. As I opened the fridge to unpack my box of provisions, which resembled a Red Cross food parcel and had been sent to me from Keith's mum Dorothy, my first impression was, 'Why is there no food in here?' That was not strictly true; I discovered a piece of unwrapped cheese, hard and cracked like the sandal injured heels of some women in summer. There was a half-eaten Mars chocolate bar and the remainder of the shelf space was filled with alcohol: cans of lager, a bottle of vodka and some half-drunk bottles of wine.

With no obvious free space for my proper food and my reluctance to move any of their items I ended up putting the wine bottles into the door of the fridge after mending the bar to hold them in place. I then squeezed my food items that needed to needed to be refrigerated into half a shelf. I turned to find a space in the cupboards above the work top for the remainder of my food. This proved to be a big mistake. There must have been some kind of alarm that triggered in their rooms announcing 'There's food in the house'. Out of nowhere they were all suddenly in the kitchen eating my food whilst eyeing up items in the box that I had yet to unpack. I placed the box on the work top and they were soon 'helping' me to sort it out into cupboards and into their mouths. Lesson learned, keep my food in my room.

At eighteen years old and living away from home for the first time I didn't appreciate how immature and naïve I was. I had always been perceived and treated as quite grown up in my little country girl world. However, here in the ancient city of Colchester, Essex a whole new world was opening up to me, and my new house mates were ready and waiting to expose me to all that it had to offer. Josie, Tracy and Karen were third year student nurses who had just taken their hospital final examinations and to any new first year students these third year students were gods. Where they went

Ooh Matron!

you followed and this journey of enlightenment has resulted in a few of the stories in this book.

Josie was a party animal who, when not in uniform, was frequently found in the local pubs and nightclubs wearing short miniskirts or Olivia Newton John, Grease style, high waist shiny trousers with the regulatory boob tube. Luckily, Josie being quite busty, it stayed in place, well most of the time! Some of her friends, less fortunate in the bust area, incurred wardrobe malfunctions at some inopportune moments, but we don't need to go into that story. Tracy the biker chick didn't go out as much, she had a hairy, long bearded boyfriend who often stayed over, despite the hospital house rules. They played their angry sounding music and drank lager.

Karen was a bit of a mystery to me and I perceived her as quite intimidating at the time. In hindsight, and now a little more worldly wise, I realise that she was a lesbian. For the first few weeks I only ever saw her dressed in her uniform. She was working night duties at Essex County Hospital and, with me on eight weeks of induction and orientation, Monday to Friday 8.30am – 5pm at the classrooms in the Severalls Hospital grounds, our paths rarely crossed. However, the first time I did see her in her out of work clothes my initial impression was that she looked or certainly dressed like a man. She never had men say over, but frequently her female 'friends' came over, with a lot of laughing, giggling and general noise for someone usually so quiet and who appeared or acted as if withdrawn from company. She always had short dyed blonde spiky hair styles and wore the Dexi's Midnight Runners style baggy dungarees with Doc Martin boots. All very fashionable at the time.

It turns out that I was considered to be extremely lucky to be allocated a room in a hospital house off campus. This privilege was usually reserved for third year students who, supposedly more responsible, would be less likely to require the discreet supervision provided by the porters at the nurses' quarters. The rest of my classmates were allocated rooms in the main block of the nurses' quarters in the hospital grounds. Their rooms were a lot smaller than my room at the house and the bathroom sharing involved a lot more forward planning.

Sarah Jane Butfield

Often after a night out in town, usually after pay-day, we all ended up being delivered in a convoy of taxis back to the nurses' quarters aiming to get ourselves in, and sometimes sneak in a guest or two. It was totally against the rules for men to sleep over. The porters would turn a blind eye if fellow students, like me, stayed over, but for male guests the rule was rigorously enforced. Nurses, however, are renowned for being resourceful, and adopting the 'where there's a will there's a way' maxim. They apparently soon found ways for boyfriends and 'new friends' made at night clubs to get into the nurses' quarters unnoticed by distracting the porters with a tasty kebab or some other food related gifts, offered by giggling, somewhat tipsy girls. However, the porters had ways to extract their revenge and they had a few cunning tricks which they utilised to flush out the forbidden male guests. I missed the funniest which involved the porters' setting off the fire alarm, usually about 3.30am in the early hours of a Friday or Saturday. They then stood with their arms folded across their chests with smug expressions on their faces as they waited to see who ran out and in what state of undress.

When my friends in the nurses' quarters first experienced this obviously they, and their male friends, got caught out. Flushed out male visitors would be told to 'be on their way', a warning given in a stern fatherly tone by the porters. However, once the first year student nurses picked up some of the tricks of the second and third year students things changed. For example, some male guests dangerously decided that when the alarm went off they would stay inside while the roll call took place outside in the car park. If there had been a real fire at any point there could well have been casualties or even fatalities, but fortunately that never happened during my time there. The other reported tool for detection involved sending the duty night sisters' in for a patrol and random spot check of the rooms. This really did sound like a scene from a carry on film like Carry on Doctor or Carry on Matron! Men in wardrobes, hidden up unused Victorian fireplaces, under beds, in the bathroom and even in the kitchen cupboards. However, the night sisters' or 'matrons' as the nurses' quarters residents called them, a team of canny, worldly wise, experienced women, were experts at finding pieces of men's clothing, shoes or boots that gave

Ooh Matron!

the game away. Once an item was found they would pursue its owner like a Rottweiler dog looking for a bone. If no one owned up then they confiscated the clothing which often led to some strangely dressed guests leaving the next morning, especially if jeans or trousers had been removed.

To be fair, the hospital houses too were subjected to 'random inspections', the term used by the porters who carried out the task, although during my time in the Mill Road house they occurred infrequently. However, Josie told me that on one occasion the Harley Davidson, parked at the front of the house in the road and always a bit of giveaway, indicated that Tracy's boyfriend Steve was in residence. Well that and the huge pair of motorcycle boots in the hallway. Although the night porters were not brave enough to ask Steve to leave, one porter did come close that night when he said, "Let's not see you here again son." But it changed nothing. Tracy, scary enough on her own, especially at night time, was in my opinion one reason we had so few inspections. This became fortuitous for me because by week four I had lost my goodie-two shoes nickname and reputation as Keith became a frequent overnight visitor at weekends when he had time off and I had work and study to do.

So here I was living away from home for the first time. I had finally upgraded from my two years at pre nursing college in Ipswich wearing my pink lady uniform, to a proper blue and white checked dress complete with white belt, hat with one blue stripe, and a black, red lined cape. For me it was a symbol of being a proper nurse and when I wore it I recalled afternoons spent with my mum watching episodes of the medical soap opera General Hospital. She loved those shows and would often talk about how she watched *Emergency Ward 10* with my Nan when she was pregnant with me or my sisters. The hats, made from stiff cardboard, came pre-marked ready for us to fold and create the correct size, with the one stripe as recognition of my training status. Student nurses wore stiff white belts that fastened at the back with hooks and eyes because no nurse buckles were permitted until you qualified. All of these status recognition factors became important to student and pupil nurses as we progressed, gaining stripes and uniform privileges in a ranking system similar to that of one of the armed forces. Worn with pride to acknowledge the work and study endured to attain the next level.

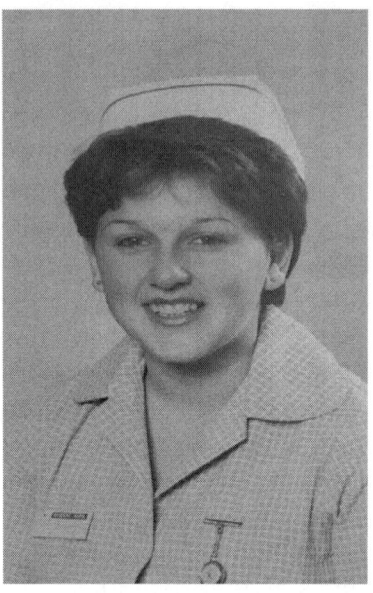

Proudly wearing my one blue stripe in my first year photograph at Colchester School of Nursing

After two months I had completed the orientation and basic skills training at the school of nursing. This included learning skills such as how to bed-bath patients unable to move unattended, a skill we practiced on each other wearing swimsuits, resulting in a great deal of giggling, laughing and general silliness. Other skills learned and practiced included the taking and recording of basic observations of body temperature, pulse, blood pressure and respiration rate, and the drawing up and administration of subcutaneous and intra muscular injections, which we practiced on blood oranges. Most importantly for first year student nurses was the skill we would use most from day one on the wards, the important art of bed making. This included forming those infamous perfectly shaped hospital corners which would be checked rigorously. My first placement as a first year student nurse would be at Severalls Hospital on my surgical allocation to Ashley Ward

Ooh Matron!

and this would be followed by eight weeks in the medical ward at Essex County Hospital before returning to the school to consolidate our learning.

Sarah Jane Butfield

Chapter three:
Banana Banshee Happy Hour

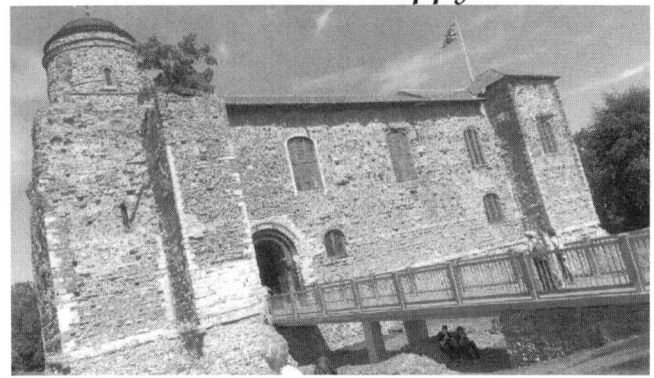

Colchester Castle 2015- Photograph courtesy of Richard Klein

Colchester has been a university town for over fifty years and has had garrison links and regiments stationed there since Roman times. The castle in Colchester was built on the foundations of the destroyed Roman Temple of Claudius. In modern times, meeting the social needs of these two large groups of people, consisting of students and squaddies, is a huge undertaking. To some people, especially local Colchester residents the term 'squaddie' would be used in the more derogatory way meaning soldiers who think they are 'God's gift to women!' As you might expect, with a large number of young and socially oriented groups of people living as part of the local community, most of the problems revolved around alcohol consumption and alcohol induced incidents. In the mid-1980s an increasing number of student nurses and trainee doctors were added into this mix as recruitment increased. The results became messy, noisy and sometimes outrageous and on pay day the town centre was always on high alert.

The October 1983 student nurse intake consisted of twenty-eight females and two males, the male nurses at that time being in the minority. However the tide was turning. Kevin and Martin in our group were good sports and didn't segregate themselves from the females who ranged in age from eighteen to forty-two.

In 1983, the pubs, bars and clubs bordering the main hospitals were always busy and in the town centre, at that time, St Mary's Hospital on Balkerne Hill and Essex County Hospital in Lexden Road provided a steady flow of staff to these drinking establishments. On the outskirts of town and closer to the nurses' quarters and my new home in Mill Road were Myland Hospital near the rugby club and Severalls Hospital near to The Dog and Pheasant pub. The Hospital Arms and various yuppie style bars in or near the High Street became popular with hospital staff of all grades.

In the 1980s after work drinks with your Filofax became increasingly popular with local business people and this bolstered the trade from the existing healthcare workers, soldiers and university students. Student nurses carried only money and emergency plasters for dancing induced blisters. As nurses and doctors worked shifts, the length of time that a night out lasted often extended into the early hours with staff adding to the numbers after each shift ended. Sometimes, on pay day, a night out lasted up to forty-eight hours. Even if we didn't have the excuse of it being pay day, groups of nurses and doctors would often meetup after their shifts to offload after a hard or taxing day. We hard working student nurses tried to confine ourselves to once a week unless a special occasion necessitated more.

In the first few months of living, working and studying in Colchester, between my fellow students and my experienced socialite housemates, I had more than my fair share of nights out on a work day. I also had my 'normal' nights out back in Suffolk when Keith took me home to catch up with my friends and family in and around Ipswich. At eighteen, fresh from college and living away from home for the first time, there was no doubt I was definitely burning the candle not just at both ends but from all other angles as well.

Student nurses received a salary when I trained although this has since changed, but getting NHS payslips for the first time evoked great pride in my new chosen career pathway. Although we all put in a lot of unpaid hours, that didn't seem to matter to any of us. Most of the jobs I had worked at during my two years at college had paid me cash in hand so to get a pay slip was a new and grown up experience.

We would go to the administration office and pick up the slim brown windowed envelopes which revealed your name and location. At the start of the day they would always be filed in alphabetical order; however, nearing the end of pay day the remaining envelopes would be out of order and sometimes out of the box and on the floor. After collecting and checking our pay packet the next task involved planning how to spend it.

There were two older women in our group and it seems a bit odd writing that now as 'an older woman' myself, but they being in their early forties, to an eighteen year old were old. These students had studied towards their State Enrolled Nurse qualification some years previously and for family or personal reasons did not complete the training. They had taken a special entrance test instead of needing the required five O levels. As they had been successful in passing the test they received a place on the SRN course to restart their studies as student nurses. They provided the motherly aspect to the group, but don't be deceived, they could party harder than some of us youngsters. Within the eighteen to twenty-one age segment, other factors also segregated our class. By this I mean those of us in relationships and those 'on the hunt'. We even had the token blonde with the perfect figure who made the uniform look wonderful. Apart from being super intelligent she intended using her student nurse years to find a suitable Registrar or Consultant to marry. That sounds so old-fashioned nowadays, but it happened then.

Learning a little from my experience in my first year at college, when I enjoyed the social life too much and did not pay enough attention to my studies, I tried to choose a safe line to walk between study and fun. Sometimes I succeeded but at other times that statement would be open for debate. I deliberately chose not to become part of the other very small segment of our group, the studious set, who rarely went out with the group and who always approached our academic tasks with relative ease when the rest of us struggled. I wasn't really in their league of intelligence anyway, so I don't think they would have welcomed me. I didn't party at every opportunity which made me feel good about my restraint and socialising choices and consequently the results I managed to achieve in my studies. Maybe I was growing up and learning from my mistakes. I made two good friends with a similar mind-set who also had long-term boyfriends: Teresa, also from Suffolk and living in the nurses' quarters, and Lorna from Colchester who lived at home with her parents. Among the socialites in our group I developed additional kudos because not only did I live in a hospital house, but I lived with Josie. Josie could get us into parties and places where 'normal first year students' would never be considered for admission.

The best of these undoubtedly were the qualified nurse parties which often occurred in the doctors' houses. Can you guess who wanted to be my new best friend? Yes, Alicia the leggy blonde, doctor hunter. By the time I was six months into my training and settling into the regime of practical placements on the wards, which were combined with two week slots in the classroom to consolidate our learning, my housemates had all qualified as State Registered Nurses. They had all been offered positions on wards at the local hospitals which meant they didn't want or need to move out for the first year. They were finished with studying, well in their eyes, which meant only one thing on their newly inflated salaries, yes you guessed it, time to socialise and party harder.

It's important to remember, before we move on, that as a born and bred country girl before arriving in the big city, (well Colchester), my drinking experience was limited. In rural Suffolk, country pubs were places to meet with friends, play darts or pool and talk. In Colchester the pubs near the hospital were often busy whatever time you visited and unless you went with friends they could be lonely places despite being crowded. The other popular hangouts, increasing in number and popularity at that time, were the trendy wine and cocktails bars, of which I had no prior experience other than what I had seen on television. I sensed I was out of place from the first visit, but the qualified nurses wanted to appear influential and these bars became the place to be seen and so where they went, there I followed.

Sarah Jane Butfield

One particular Friday night we were in a bar opposite Essex County Hospital, we hadn't made it far! I don't remember exactly what we were celebrating, probably just finishing work, but anyway we seemed set for a long night. We knew this because Josie had a handbag with her. This always indicated a long night laid ahead and that she was prepared in case she might need to go straight to work in the morning from town! The bag contained the essentials: underwear, replacement makeup, Paracetamol, Pro-plus caffeine tablets, her belt and fob watch. She left her shoes and spare uniform at work for such occasions.

That night a lot of new faces in town meant a new regiment had arrived at the garrison, which always increased the excitement of the 'man hunters' in our party. Squaddies were easy to spot even out of uniform. There's a stereotypical image and they lived up to it rigorously. The regulation short haircut, a muscular, fit physique and the pride to show it off with the squaddie swagger. This swagger was always more pronounced when they walked in a group which meant 'the boys are back in town, so look out'. Fighting outside pubs and clubs was commonplace, but unavoidable, like most garrison towns where squaddies and local lads usually ended up fighting over a woman or a spilt drink.

Lorna's boyfriend was in the army, and she took a lot of ribbing about it, as people who didn't know her often assumed it was a fling while he was stationed there. However, he was Colchester born and bred. She didn't feel comfortable with the group we were out with on this particular night and she went home before happy hour got underway in the bar. Happy hour, oh why do they call it that? It might cause your bank balance to be happy during the hour of cheap drinks, but the after effects do not always incite happy memories.

Happy hour in the wine bar meant lounging on a mix of sofas, arranged to replicate a trendy person's apartment. However, being situated in the body of an old building and overlooking the busy Lexden Road traffic lights, it didn't really have the desired effect on me. After a full eight hour shift at the hospital, relaxing into the sofas after one drink was far too easy and dangerous because I could settle myself in for the night or even fall asleep. That said, when we were there specifically for happy hour it all worked very

Ooh Matron!

differently. The idea or plan was to drink as much as possible during happy hour so that we would not need to buy as many drinks when the prices returned to normal. The plan whenever we visited wine or cocktail bars for happy hour was that one person would choose the drink and we would all drink that cocktail for the entire hour. Tonight the cocktail of choice was the banana banshee. I had never heard of it and when the first one arrived it looked like a small milkshake in a wide topped glass. Since I don't drink milk, I was immediately put off from drinking it.

I remember thinking when I took the first tentative sip that it didn't taste as if it contained any alcohol. With this misconception firmly planted in my subconscious, I began drinking freely, much too freely, especially as we had now attracted some uninvited male attention and they were buying the cocktails for us. This apparently common trick would supposedly make them look generous to the women they bought drinks for and who they hoped would keep them company for the remainder of the evening and possibly the night. Of course they never considered that we could be clever enough to work out that they were only generous during happy hour when cheap cocktails were available. Knowing that they assumed that all girls are easily impressed by flash men who generously buy lots of drinks, we let them keep thinking that and overindulged at their expense. The extremely sweet tasting viscous drink, which had a banana odour and pale colour, bore no other resemblance to a drink, it actually resembled a dessert. We seemed to be able to drink them in three or four mouthfuls because they were smooth, small and increasingly tasty. However, because of this they made us thirsty and we needed to drink more.

When happy hour finished we knew the time had come to move on. The drink buying males had become annoying and far too touchy feely for my liking. Josie didn't want them following us around either as it might hinder her chances with a real man that night. When they realised we weren't interested the atmosphere and their moods changed and the more sober members of our party decided our time was up in this bar. With happy hour over we headed for the next watering hole, quite literally called The Hole in the Wall, a pub on Balkerne Hill.

Although some local residents believed the name of the pub to be related to the destruction of the walled defences around Colchester by Boudicca in 60 AD in fact the name originates from a premeditated hole being made in the wall of the pub when it was called the Kings Head.

"In 1843, the owners of the Kings Head had part of the roman wall, outside, demolished in order to insert a new window overlooking the new railway station. This led to the pub being nicknamed the "Hole in the Wall". The nickname remained until 1963 when the pub was officially renamed the Hole in the Wall." Courtesy of *http://pubshistory.com/EssexPubs/Colchester/kinghead.shtml*

As we left the hot, stuffy atmosphere in the cocktail bar and my face met the fresh, cool, evening air outside two things started to happen. First my stomach started churning and I developed a watery sensation in my mouth as a build-up of saliva increased. I knew what this meant. I was imminently going to be sick. Secondly, either I had double or blurred vision or the size of our party had increased enormously since we exited the cocktail bar. Josie must have noticed my green around the gills complexion because she quickly ushered me to the side of the road in case the sickness could not be contained.

"We will soon be at the pub, don't worry," she said.

At that moment another pub or bar was the last place I wanted to go, but being physically incapable of going anywhere on my own, with Josie's assistance I continued on. Living in a house often full of Josie's party animal friends, I had seen and heard the stories of tricks and tips for being able to party all night without being sick or forgetting where you lived. Some of the tales they told about situations they had got themselves into would make your eyes roll and your head shake in disbelief, but on this particular night out I was about to experience one of the proven party all night remedies first hand.

When we arrived at the next pub, Josie placed something in my hand that resembled a piece of soft rubber and escorted me to the toilets. As I entered the cubicle I opened my hand to reveal an already unwrapped suppository. I knew what it was as we had already started learning about them and administering them during our training, but hey I'm not constipated, so what's this all about? I opened the door and my look of bewilderment must have said it all.

"Just do it," she said, "it will make you feel better and I ain't goin home yet."

I didn't have the mental capability to argue or investigate further, as the intensity of the desire to vomit increased by the second. So I did as instructed and inserted the suppository. I found out afterwards that carrying antiemetic (anti-sickness) suppositories was standard kit for an all-nighter. As much as I didn't want to admit it, within fifteen minutes the nausea abated and I hadn't been sick. After composing myself over a glass of lemonade and lime cordial which Josie assured everyone was vodka, in no time at all I resumed drinking vodka and lime with the rest of the party. I have never repeated this treatment and I would not recommend it. I never did know or dared to ask where from or how she acquired her party first aid medicines, but that night I was grateful for it.

Chapter four:
Mind your backs!

How many names or titles can be given to one aspect of training? Over the years, the methodology of moving patients, lifting and moving equipment and facilitating patient independence during episodes of immobility has changed enormously. The majority of the change has been driven by knowledge, injury to healthcare staff and patients and increased technological advances. Some examples include:

- Lifting and Handling
- Manual Handling
- Moving and Handling
- Safer transfer of people and objects and the list goes on.

When I started my training I thought I knew how to lift objects such as boxes, pieces of furniture and other people's children. At home and in various work roles such as babysitter, fruit picker, waitress, barmaid and so on I had needed to lift and so I did. However, in college, when I received my first formal training in what was then called lifting and handling, I realised how little I knew about the impact of incorrect lifting technique and posture in relation to the safety of myself and my patients.

Even though we were not insured and thus not permitted to take part in manoeuvres that resulted in the patient being lifted or raised from a surface such as a bed or chair, we could assist with mobility transfers, as long as the patient could stand and bear their own weight. I didn't realise at that time, due to my inexperience, that these manoeuvres can be more dangerous than lifting as a pair or in a team. This is because, for a variety of reasons patients can just collapse from a presumably safe standing position. An example of this would be if the patient experienced a drop in their blood pressure after sitting or lying for extended periods. The act of standing up, after prolonged sitting, is enough to cause this condition, which is often referred to as postural hypotension. This happens because the position change temporarily reduces the blood flow and consequently oxygen to the brain. This leads to feelings of light-headedness and, sometimes, fainting and/or loss of consciousness.

As part of my lifting and handling induction and training as a first year student nurse I was first introduced to the Australian Lift. It was commonly used for stroke patients as it meant that you carried the weight through their armpit and your shoulder therefore reducing the pressure and strain on their limbs, especially important in those with paralysis.

Here is a definition of the Australian Lift:
Courtesy of http://medical-dictionary.thefreedictionary.com/Australian+lift

"A type of shoulder lift used to move a patient who is unable to assume a sitting position on a bed or other surface. The lift is executed by two persons, one on each side of the patient who place their shoulders near the patient under the patient's axillae. At the same time, the two lifters grasp each other's hands under the patient's thighs and make coordinated movements needed to lift the patient onto or from a bed or wheelchair."

If you are interested in seeing this lift in action and finding out more about the safety issues you might enjoy this link.
https://www.youtube.com/watch?v=WJ2aocvZg0I

The three other physical lifting techniques taught at that time were:

The Orthodox Lift – often referred to as a two-person lift, where each nurse places one arm around the patient's back and their other arm under the patient's thighs. The nurses then clasp each other's wrists to lift the patient.

Next The Drag Lift - There were a few variations on this now banned lift, which consisted of two nurses, each taking hold of an arm and a leg and then lifting the patient up in the bed or out and into a chair.

Finally; The Bear Hug – this was the move of choice taught to enable a nurse to single-handedly pick up and transfer a patient from the edge of the bed into a chair or vice versa. The nurse would stand in front of the patient placing the patient's arms around her neck whilst she clasped her arms in a bear hug type hold around the patient's torso, clasping her wrists at the back, or if a handling belt was worn, by holding the handles at the back and then using her body weight to pivot the patient up and around to the new place to sit.

These lifts are no longer permitted for health and safety reasons, not only for nurses but also for patients. However, given the names and the range of positions that amateurs at these lifts would find themselves in, you can probably imagine some of the shenanigans that occurred during our practice sessions. Our practical sessions always involved us taking turns at being the patient. With the exception of practicing bed baths and the use of the bath sling, when we needed to wear a swimsuit, we were permitted to wear tracksuit trousers and a tee shirt instead of our uniforms for practical lifting classes. This always seemed ridiculous to me, because on the wards we would be wearing our uniforms and would be restricted by the inflexible dress material, our stockings, hats and belts not to mention the problems of the rising skirt as we conducted these manoeuvres. Plus have you ever seen a nurse without a pocket full of pens, scissors and pieces of paper?

On one such training session I was the patient and my role was to pretend to be a patient who had a right below knee amputation and whose condition was complicated by a sacral pressure sore. Hmm… nice! My colleagues had to plan and execute the move to get me from a hospital bed into an inappropriate geriatric ward armchair. Their remit was that they needed to position me comfortably and safely. The chair would have been more at home in a retirement home and was unfit for purpose, but then that was the aim of this little test. How would they navigate the height difference and the arms that are not removable? With a big white dressing pad stuck to the outside of my tracksuit trousers on my sacral area to indicate the location of the pressure sore, and a pillow case placed over my foot and fastened with tape below my right knee to indicate the amputated limb, I laid on my back on the bed. I knew that I looked funny because the class were already laughing before Mandy and Julie even attempted to move me. They elected to use

Ooh Matron!

the Australian Lift so that they could clasp hands under both my thighs thus accommodating the amputated leg area. After pulling me, rather roughly as I recall, into a sitting position, they manoeuvred me to the edge of the bed. Now at this point if my pressure sore had been real it would have been exposed and extremely painful because they totally disregarded it as they dragged me and caused the dressing to come away.

Once at the edge of the bed they started to position themselves on either side to enable them to place their shoulders under my armpits. Unfortunately, they were not the same height and Mandy, a mere 5ft tall (152.5cm), had to climb onto the bed beside me and Julie, who was nearer to 5ft 7in (170 cm), crouched down. This meant one of my armpits was being forced higher than the other to accommodate them. Our precarious set up was destined for failure and this state of imbalance meant that, as they tilted me back to position their hands under my thighs, all three of us fell backwards onto the bed and they ended up laying on both of my arms. Mr Waters, our tutor rushed over, but was laughing so much he couldn't speak. I am so grateful I trained in the age before mobile phones and Facebook as that image would have been circulated very quickly. Once we had all regained our composure and I retook my position with a replacement pretend dressing applied, Mr Waters talked everyone through the mistakes they made, including the initial one of not realising that they were an incompatible lifting team.

The other concept that changed during my training and continues to be adapted is the counting mechanism. It always has been fraught with danger due to miscommunication and human error. When a nurse says we go on three, does that mean you count one, two and then lift on three? Or do you count one, two, three and then lift? That split second of difference can result in a neck or back injury or the patient being dropped. The same inconsistency can be applied to ready, steady, go. By the end of my training in 1986 it was one, two, three, lift and you lifted and moved the patient on the word lift.

As the incidence of neck and back injuries among healthcare staff and in particular nurses continued to increase over the years, the introduction and need for mechanised lifting aids became big business as did the training of staff in their use.

'In the NHS, manual handling accidents accounted for 52% of all sickness absence.' Ref: Manual Handling Operations Regulations 1993 amended 2002

'The total annual cost to the NHS is 400 million pounds per year, enough to employ16,000 nurses.' Ref: Back Care 2011 (Cited Nursing Times)

According to the Royal College of Nursing: *'1.5 million working days are lost every year because of back injuries to nurses. 80% of nurses have time off with back problems each year; 3600 healthcare workers are forced to retire early as a result of back injury.'* (Back Care (cited Nursing Times 2011))

You will read more about moving and handling changes in education and practice later in the series as I tackle this hands on as a nurse educator.

Again due to lack of life experience in those early days, I assumed that the reasons for immobility would be led by physical and predominantly medical conditions. However, a large amount of immobility was exacerbated by weight issues and as the obesity problems around the world continued to increase so did the size of the patients we cared for. When I was first introduced to the term bariatric, for some unknown reason in my mind it sounded like a piece of diving equipment or a method of measurement like a barometer. My family still laugh at me when I remind them that medical terminology does not always follow a logical route in my brain.

The term bariatric means the area of medicine that handles obesity and its associated disease processes using the control and treatment of body weight. In 1983 the range of bariatric lifting equipment was not as extensive as it is now and it was not widely available in the NHS. There was little in the way of specially adapted or oversized wheelchairs and commodes, etc., therefore many lifting and moving issues stemmed from large patients getting wedged into equipment and places that made it difficult and dangerous to get them out of. Many a time we had to climb onto patient's bed to physically reposition them onto their sides or onto a slide board, which is undignified for staff and patients alike.

The equipment we used in the 1980s was considered mainstream and unless specially adapted it made no distinction for the weight and size of the patient. There was simply an adult or paediatric sling for the hoists. Now they come in sizes ranging from paediatric XXS to XXL for up to 500lb adults. Then we move into bariatric slings ranging M to XXL managing weights from 300lb to 1000lbs. They are all complete with colour coding and special materials for bathing slings, etc. The other major change in the equipment was the transition from manual devices to battery or electric operated devices. My first hoist experience was with an Oxford hoist which looked like something from a mechanics workshop. During our induction period we had to practice on each other being hoisted from the bed to a chair. The pain and scrapes from the incorrectly applied hoisting slings and the chaffing from, what was then acceptable, crossing of the leg straps if you were too small and at risk of falling out, always made me extra careful when I began using them on patients on the wards. Fortunately the 1980s was a time of intense research and development and new and improved equipment and hoists, as well as regulations on the amount of space needed to operate hoists, progressed rapidly. The biggest obstacle to the advance towards safe practice was that a large proportion of hospitals in the NHS were built long before hospital hoists were first invented and put into service in the late 1950s and early 1960s. Consequently, many corridors and doorways were not wide enough to accommodate the regular use of hoisting equipment.

The next lifting or movement aids which caused a lot of hilarity when we were learning how to use them were slide and banana boards. Why were they called banana boards? Simply because of their shape, slightly curved and the fact that the majority of them were yellow. Even the name of that second one conjures up comedic images of patients sliding on bananas. Let me explain. The slide board is a straight piece of plastic carefully moulded with rounded edges and tapered ends to allow a patient to transfer from a wheelchair to their bed or vice versa. They could also be used for wheelchair to toilet transfers. The curved banana transfer boards made transfers around fixed objects such as armrest and chair-arms safer and more accessible.

To begin with, some of equipment names sounded like jokes to us as students learning this new language not only of anatomy and physiology but also of equipment. It took a little while for the seriousness to overcome the laughter, innuendo and hilarity that some of our training session involved. I mean, we moved from banana boards to monkey poles. Didn't we all play on those in the park as kids, hanging and swinging around? But here, in the nursing world, monkey poles were attached to the beds of patients who could use their upper limbs and body strength to move or reposition themselves up in the bed unaided. These were particularly useful for the orthopaedic patients with legs in plaster casts or bolted into weighted traction. From bananas to monkeys, there was so much to learn and become familiar with before we were let loose on patients, but we did have a lot of fun.

After establishing the basics we would move onto ward based lifting and handling tuition from trained nurses and the auxiliary nurses which included the use of lifting belts, unorthodox drawsheet manoeuvres, slide sheets and the adaptation of the lifts we had been shown in our orientation training. Adaptations which were practical but which our tutors would have frowned upon.

Chapter five:
Slip, slop, slap summer fun

As the first year of training entered the summer months of 1984 our house became an even more popular hangout and we reaped the benefits of this in many ways. We were fortunate to have a big garden with full maintenance provided by the hospital gardeners and we made good use of it. These large semi-detached houses, originally built for growing families, frequently became shared residences in university towns and cities. Ours, sub-divided and with the addition of wash basins in each room, enabled students and nurses, who initially were strangers to each other, to cohabit with a degree of independence. Nonetheless, due to its design, the bonus was that it still provided great entertainment spaces for its occupants and their guests. With a large area of lawn and a barbeque area, the garden soon became known as 'party central'. Friends who lived in the nurses' quarters popped round before late or night shifts to sunbathe. All visitors and their guests brought gifts of cakes, biscuits or fruit juices if they came before work, alcohol, snacks and barbeque food if they came after work. We didn't buy food all summer, but the normally sparsely occupied shelves became fully laden with left over salad items, cooked burgers, sausages and chicken. Of course, any alcohol not consumed came into our ownership by default, retained for future use.

One sunny, hot afternoon I came home after an early shift, about 3.30pm, looking forward to a few hours in the garden catching up on my surgical case study assignment. As I approached the house I noticed the front door was wide open. This unusual sight immediately triggered alarm bells with me because one of the rigorously enforced house rules was never to leave it open and always to use the back door to let in fresh air as we could not see or hear if people walked in the front door if we were in our rooms. Josie's room, the only one with clear view if occupied was a wasted resource as she couldn't be relied on. She slept for long periods especially in day time due to shift work and socialising. I entered the house and looked down the hall through the kitchen and in the garden I could see a group of four people scantily dressed, well pretty much naked. I didn't recognise any of them and I did not see any of my house mates indoors or out accompanying them. It is important to remember, as it is very different now, that at this time no one had personal mobile phones, the first one only introduced in 1985. In addition, living in a shared house, we had no landline telephone and the nearest public telephone box was situated along Mill Road approximately 500 yards away. Without thinking, of my personal safety, I closed the front door behind me and walked through the hall towards the kitchen. As I got closer I did momentarily think, 'What the hell are you doing'? However, I carried on regardless and as bravery engulfed me or during this moment of naïve stupidity I opened the back door and walked into the garden. The four people, three women and one man, all turned to look at me as if I was the intruder.

"Can we help you?" The man, wearing just some skimpy swim trunks, said.

I was really angry now.

"I think you mean, can I help you? This is my home, what the hell are you doing?"

"I think you are mistaken, this is my sister's house," he said.

At this point all four of them, now standing with their arms folded across their scantly clothed chests made me feel outnumbered. I tried to maintain an assertive stance as I found myself shaking as the adrenaline fight or flight reaction kicked in although I wasn't really sure that they presented a threat to me. Seriously, would they be a threat to me, wearing swim wear? It became quite hard to take them seriously, I sensed myself smirk, which then developed into a smile spreading across my face, and after all I was the one in uniform. The smile must have angered them as they looked at each other, started whispering and their confident facial expressions deserted them.

"And your sister is who exactly?"

The man rolled his eyes and turned towards his friends, "Sorry ladies".

Then just as he turned his attention back to me, a loud familiar voice bellowed from the kitchen.

Ooh Matron!

"Janey, you've met my brother. He's handsome isn't he?" Josie said, adding a big wink of her right eye with an emphasised head movement, one of her trademark mannerisms. Josie. Of course he had to be related to Josie, the resemblance obvious now. The extrovert stance, minimal clothing, surrounded by members of the opposite sex; why I didn't work that out for myself.

Janey, my nickname amongst my housemates, wasn't popular with my boyfriend. He liked just plain Sarah, always one to keep things simple. He also did not like the fact that I lived with housemates older than me who exerted 'a bad influence on me'. This in itself was pure irony as Keith was eleven years my senior and my mum had said that he had been a bad influence on me since we met and fell in love when I was fifteen and him being twenty-six. Funny that.

Joseph, or Jo to the ladies, Josie's brother, had been invited down for the weekend and Josie had left them a key, but obviously not the house rule instructions about leaving the door open.

In the 1980s the danger of sunburn or sun damage to your skin and general health was not as widely publicised or documented as it is now. Everyone saw the adverts for sunscreen, but as the sun in the UK was unreliable and often absent for days at a time in summer, when the sun did come out so did the array of bodies on our lawn. Jugs of drinks filled our fridge and our ice box became home to a secret weapon against party poopers or killjoys. Of course, the first one to be caught out by the trick was the naïve country girl, me. The first of my mistakes was the announcement that I intended to go into the garden to study when we already had garden party guests in residence. The second, accepting a drink from Josie. She made me a cold drink to take with me to my quiet shaded area of the garden, away from the guests. An innocent looking orange juice and lemonade with ice. I should have remembered that Josie doesn't make drinks for anyone, she liked to be waited on. I sat studying and drinking and she kept my glass topped up. Before long I decided to 'take a break' to join everyone on the lawn. They were all laughing and fooling around and then the next thing I remembered was waking up with my face under a book. As I went to move the book from my face the pain in my hands and arms was excruciating. I tossed my head to remove the book and with bleary eyes looked down at my arms. To call them sunburnt would be a massive understatement. The bright red appearance did not reflect the level of pain being experienced or the fact that they were too painful to bend or move and definitely could not be touched. Looking around I realised that the party guests had gone and it must now be evening time as the sun was low in the sky. As I struggled to get up without using my arms, more pain attacked me, this time from my feet. I had been wearing a pair of culottes so my legs had been exposed from mid-calf down and they too were burnt.

As I sat there on the grass, Karen came out from the kitchen and burst into fits of laughter before realising that I actually needed some help. She manoeuvred me into a standing position, but my feet were sore on the soles as well, although not as bad as the rest of my feet. To find a positive note in all of this, my trademark nurses' hard skin on my big toes and heels had protected my feet a little from being completely burnt. Once indoors, Karen got some wet towels and sat me at the kitchen table with a cold drink. I looked at the drink that she poured from the jug in the fridge.

"It's not very cold, but probably best you don't have any more of the ice today. It looks like you had enough to drink already."

Feeling really quite unwell and in pain I did not understand what she meant or alluded to with her comments. I had been studying and drinking orange juice and lemonade. I couldn't stomach the drink and opted for a glass of water even though I don't like drinking water. So what had happened? Well, it turned out that the ice in my drinks had been vodka ice flakes and they were the reason for the abandonment of my studying and my ending up prone on the grass with an open book on my face. Actually I was grateful for the book. Otherwise my face too would have been scorched. We had trays of this mixture in the freezer which were broken up into ice flakes, really good with a gin and tonic.

The simple aim of the ice flakes was to get the non-drinkers into the summer garden party mood. It's so wrong, but when you are not the victim it's kind of right as well if you know what I mean. I

Ooh Matron!

must confess though we probably caused some visitors to risk being caught for drink driving that summer. Bad Sarah Jane.

The other big incident that occurred that summer was when the Harley Davidson went missing! It was regularly parked outside our house and clearly indicated that Tracy had company. When that happened you did not disturb her or them. No sign on the door needed for her, unlike Josie who would stick up pieces of paper with Micropore surgical tape, sometimes even writing the name of her guest on it. I think the bike incident originated from the use of the vodka ice flakes because I am sure no one would have been brave enough to touch the Harley Davidson if they were sober. Well, except for Keith who accidently knocked it over one morning when he was taking me to work on an early shift. However, he managed to upright it and luckily, there being no damage, we escaped punishment. Anyway I digress. So on this particular Friday evening, a small group of nurses arrived at our house to plan a holiday to Spain with Josie. They took over the kitchen and worked their way through all available food and drinks. They were not supposed to be drinking, as all of them except two had early shifts the next day and therefore needed to get home that evening. The noise levels increased and suddenly around 11.30pm it all went quiet. Thinking no more of it at the time, I was soon asleep. Next morning, hoping to have a lay in as I was on a late shift not starting until 1.30pm, I was awoken by heavy knocking on my door. Opening the door in my pyjamas I was quite alarmed to find Tracy's biker boyfriend standing there in his motorcycle leather trousers, frayed denim jacket covered by a leather sleeveless over jacket adorned with a patchwork of badges.

"Did you hear them?"

"Who? What?" I said, still half asleep maybe even dreaming, I hoped.

"The thieving toe rags who nicked my bike!"

"Oh god, no sorry. Why? When did it happen?"

He didn't reply, he simply turned and thundered down the stairs in his heavy biker boots. I quickly got dressed and went downstairs to find out what was happening. He was pacing the street looking left and right as Tracy sat on the bottom stair tread swearing while putting her boots on.

"We're off to the cop shop," she said, "if you see Josie tell her I wanna talk to her."

They left heading towards Turner Road. I had never seen him walk any distance before other than around the house or out to his motorbike parked in the road. He had a strange stance and towered above Tracy in way I had previously never noticed. No one came back before I set off for work and when I returned home at 10pm the full story of the missing Harley Davidson started to be revealed as the shouting continued between Josie and Karen. Apparently one of Josie's friends, in a moment of madness presumably, thought it would be funny to move the Harley Davidson to the side of the house out of sight. Neither Tracy or her boyfriend found this funny, and it turns out neither did the police when they came to the house that evening to see where the bike had been stolen from only to find the bike on the path that leads to the back garden. Tracy and Josie did not speak to each other for several weeks and the Harley Davidson didn't stay over as often either.

Chapter six:
Wacky races and sad faces

An eight week placement on the female geriatric ward at St Mary's Hospital, after the thrills and spills of working in the extremely busy and stimulating medical and surgical wards did not sound very appealing to me, even though care of the elderly had been one of my original reasons for pursuing my career path. As a first year student nurse, eager to get in and stay in the cut and thrust of hospital action and adventure, I wanted to see, learn and experience everything. Then just when I had got into the swing of it, all I was assigned to was routine rounds of turning immobile patients, some of them suffering from horrendous pressure sores or, if I was even more unlucky, collecting and cleaning endless bedpans.

The first week dragged, as I failed to see what we could possibly learn in this slow, uneventful, routine led environment. However, by week two, with a patient selected for my case study on rehabilitation after a stroke or Cerebrovascular Accident (CVA), I settled into the ward routine and decided to make the most of my time there. The staff on the ward were extremely friendly and were hilarious to work with. The morale was high and they loved having students working on the ward because it injected them with a renewed motivation to share and expand their knowledge. Contrary to my initial thoughts, there was a great deal to learn, not least how to take responsibility. With staffing levels considerably lower than the other wards I had worked on, students were allocated patients of their own. This meant that each student nurse became responsible for all aspects of their patients' care, with the added importance of efficiently and correctly using the physical support of the auxiliary nurses and the medical knowledge and mentoring expertise of the junior staff nurses on the ward. It was mind boggling yet exhilarating to talk to newly qualified staff nurses about the second and third years of the registered nurse training and I found it inspirational to hear how many students passed their finals on the first attempt.

In elderly care, although the patients had an underlying medical reason for being an in-patient in hospital, there was deservedly a huge emphasis on maintaining their psychological well-being in the hospital environment, being separated from family, friends and loved ones, including their pets. Although a relatively new concept in 1984, the idea of allowing dogs to visit their owners, or having specially trained dogs visit either in the hospital grounds or very occasionally in the day room on the ward, began to be being trialled. There had been a new charity founded in 1983 called 'Pets As Therapy' which started spreading the word, explaining the rationale behind the scheme to rehabilitation centres, social workers and occupational therapists in a variety of healthcare arenas including hospitals. They had quickly identified that elderly care would be an ideal starting point for the project. As a dog lover, and missing having a pet of my own whilst living in the nurse's accommodation, I enjoyed finding out more about this project and soon discovered how rewarding and stimulating it could be for the patients, their families and the staff.

Working in any non-acute area gives rise to staff entertaining themselves during quiet periods, such as when patients were encouraged to rest after lunch before visiting times, etc. This time for the staff was supposed to be spent doing the special ward deep cleaning jobs such as dismantling and cleaning the wheelchairs which, although rather tedious, was one of the more appealing deep cleaning jobs. At weekends the deep cleaning schedule focused on the sluice room and the commodes and this was never popular.

The wheelchair antics started very innocuously. Jo, one of the auxiliary nurses mentioned that when she had completed her induction into working at St Mary's Hospital, one of the first things that she had to do was to push another new auxiliary nurse around in wheelchair. The aim was for them to experience the feeling of vulnerability that patients can get when they are out of control and being pushed between departments or around the ward. We had completed something similar, or so I thought, during our orientation when my training first started. However, it quickly became apparent that the ward based training in wheelchair driving was more robust than that in the school of nursing classroom situation. I volunteered to be the patient expecting a gentle tour of the hospital and the grounds, as supposedly we would be going to practice the transition from hospital floor surfaces to tarmac driveway. Well, I certainly experienced that. On the ward, in view of the ward sister, who was familiar with wheelchair training using the students as guinea pigs, the auxiliary nurse pushed me quite sedately, but the moment we hit the corridor it was if I had been shot from a cannon. I wasn't strapped in and I screamed as if riding on a roller coaster. Jo said, "Be quiet will you, the best is yet to come." In reality we couldn't have been going very fast as Jo was a big girl who didn't usually have a fast gear. That said, I certainly did feel vulnerable sitting in the wheelchair. As we approached the door to the gardens we slowed and the feeling of relief gave me a false sense of security that this experience would soon be over. I eagerly awaited the opportunity to get out even if it meant I had to push Jo and her heavy frame back to the ward. As we approached the door she spun the chair round so that she could push open the door with her voluptuous bottom, which meant I was now travelling in reverse. As the cool air from outside met the back of my head my nurses hat flapped as the hairgrips which held it in place loosened. I grabbed hold of my hat releasing my grip on the wheelchair just as she tilted the chair back onto two wheels to get it over the small step in the doorway. The feeling of moving and leaning backwards was the final straw in this learning experience and I pushed myself forward, landing in the doorway just as Jo, who now had an empty wheelchair, landed on her bottom with the chair on top of her. The sense of relief when she started laughing was immense, but in all seriousness it could have been a disaster if she had been injured or if we had broken the wheelchair. How would we have explained that? The big problem now, we both had huge holes and ladders in our uniform black tights. Punk rocker girls would have been proud to wear these tights, but we still had three hours of our shift to work with no opportunity to go and change or get replacements. There would be some explaining to do on our return to the ward. However, the story of our wacky races calamity caused staff room laughs for the remainder of my time at

St Mary's as the story was retold time and time again. Thank goodness there was no Facebook or mobile phones around then or I suspect the whole world would have had evidence of it.

As in life, where there is happiness there is also sadness. The sad side of geriatric care is not about bereavement or grief; instead it's about heartache and the pressure on families when an elderly family member suffers a stroke or an accident. This pressure is increased when the condition causes the patient to lose the ability to mobilise safely or to be able to live independently at home. A large number of patients had extended stays in the female geriatric ward, not because they needed ongoing medical observation or treatment, but because there were insufficient resources available to them within the community to facilitate their return home. I found it heartbreaking to see elderly couples prised apart by life changing medical conditions, some of which I knew would result in them being permanently separated by eventual death. The female patient who I chose for my total patient care assessment case study was a good example. She had suffered a stroke and had been stabilised on the medical ward at Essex County Hospital before being transferred to St Mary's Hospital for her aftercare and transition home. Aftercare for a stroke in her case was a course of anti-coagulant therapy, as her stroke was diagnosed as being the result of a blood clot in her brain. This is one of the commonest causes of stroke as it is usually associated with high blood pressure, hardening and blocking of the arteries with plaque which slows down the blood and allows clots to form. The fatty plaque deposits build up inside the arteries over time causing damage to the artery walls, which in turn allows clots to form. When the clot obstructs the blood flow to a particular area of the brain, inevitably some temporary or permanent damage occurs, and the physical presentation of a stroke takes place in the form of paralysis, loss of speech, memory impairment, etc. The plaque and fragments of the clots can also travel to the brain from other areas of the body. Most strokes are the result of atherosclerosis (plaque formation) and high blood pressure (hypertension) or both, which can be caused by smoking and raised cholesterol levels among other things.

The medical treatment for my patient consisted of the then standard protocol: she underwent stabilisation on twice daily subcutaneous heparin injections into the fatty layer of her abdomen, before commencing warfarin tablet therapy, (blood thinning treatment,) and she had regular blood tests to establish the correct dosage for her blood composition. This was combined with a regular small daily dose of aspirin as a preventative measure for the long-term, because although aspirin is an analgesic it also thins the blood and helps prevent new clots forming.

However, resolving and treating the physical effects of a stroke is only one part of the holistic care package needed, and the additional psychological and emotional aspects piqued my interest in elderly care. My patient, who we will call Joan, was sixty-eight years old and married to a wonderfully devoted man. I don't know his exact age, but I would say he was also in his late sixties. He visited every day, despite not being in the best of health himself. He suffered from arthritis which restricted his movements and because his wife, who was his carer, was now in hospital he relied heavily on his daughter to bring him to visit Joan and to care for him at home. The future for them was very uncertain as their daughter had a young family of her own and it was impossible to say how much physical improvement Joan would make, if any. Her stroke had affected the left side of her brain, which meant she had a right sided weakness (paralysis) and impaired speech, which added to the frustrations for both of them. Over the remaining weeks of my placement on the geriatric ward Joan had physiotherapy and occupational therapy assessments to establish what level of care and support she would need at home or in an aged care establishment. Then they had to arrange a home assessment visit for her husband to establish his needs, independently of Joan's. When I left the ward my case study closed with the sentence: 'The future for Joan is yet to be decided and may well involve a temporary or permanent stay in a nursing home, but ultimately they could end up in residential care together.' This was a very sad sentence to write and it made the case study appear incomplete. There was no ta-dah happy ending or even a conclusion as there had been in my medical ward practice case study on diabetes. In that case the patient had been diagnosed, stabilised and discharged on a regime of medication and blood monitoring which would be managed at home by the patient, their doctor and district nurse team.

The vulnerability and sadness of old age suddenly became glaringly obvious to me, as a young woman whose grandmother died when I was in my early teens, with no aging relatives to relate this experience to. I couldn't get Joan and her situation out of my thoughts and I visited her for weeks after my placement finished. Sadly, Joan died in St Mary's Hospital and her husband, who by that time was in residential care himself as his family were unable to cope, died a few weeks later. I had heard about elderly people who supposedly died of a broken heart, but working in the medical profession, where there has to be a physical reason for someone to die, the concept was hard for me to accept until this happened. The sadness on his face as he walked into the ward became hidden behind a forced yet loving smile every minute that he sat at Joan's bedside holding her hand. The image is engrained on my soul and the memory of it is as vivid today as it was real then. The pressure on spouses, when their soul mate becomes not only physically separated from them by hospitalisation or the transfer to an aged care facility, but sometimes physically changed by accident, illness or age-related deterioration is immense. In 1984 there was much less support available to families who even considered nursing or caring for family members at home. Now, although aged care provision is continually in high demand, the allied healthcare support services have grown and developed to accommodate the increasing demands of our ageing population. When I reflect now on the path of my nursing career I know that this experience with Joan and her husband may have played a subconscious part in some of my career decisions, because care of the elderly became one of the most rewarding areas of healthcare that I ever worked in. Elderly people who are not in denial about their condition or abilities are on the whole so grateful for the input of all grades of staff in whatever healthcare establishment they find themselves. Taking the time to listen to them and taking the holistic approach to their physical, psychological and social care needs helped me to develop not only as nurse, but also as an adult in a world where our history is often held in the minds of these frail people, some of whom fought wars and personal battles to protect future generations.

Chapter seven:
Do I really want to be a nurse?

The second year as a student nurse saw the workload, assessments and study increase to become a testing time. Our tutors had joked about the 'two stripe blues' in our first year, but as a keen and eager beginner I convinced myself that it would never happen to me. I would call it a mid-point crisis, a bit like a midlife crisis now that I have experienced both and can compare notes.

Things started to change and at the time I didn't realise how easily little pieces of my life veered off uncontrollably in different directions. From a professional viewpoint I had moved into a year of specialist ward placements which included ophthalmic surgery, gynaecology, obstetrics and psychiatry. Written down like that it looks like an even stranger mix than I perceived it at the time. I had no interest in eye care whatsoever. I struggled to administer my own chloramphenicol ointment when I had conjunctivitis and so the thought of touching and being responsible for the eye care of children and adults at Myland Hospital hung over me like a dark cloud. My time in the ophthalmic specialist unit was a surgical allocation and would form part of my 760 hours of surgical practical experience during my three years training. It would include working in the operating theatres, out-patient clinic, day-case surgery and ward based pre and post-operative care. In the two weeks before I started, when we did our introduction to ophthalmic nursing in the classroom, I struggled to take it all in. I think I was so nervous about the placement my brain just would not acknowledge any further information about eyes. The eye is such a delicate, crucial organ and I became consumed by self-doubt and low confidence. I loved nursing, but I suddenly felt inadequate and I hadn't even started yet.

After studying the history of nursing on my pre nursing course, the history of Myland Hospital fascinated me. In the late 1800s, as a farm, it formed part of the Severalls estate at the end of Mill Road. Its location made it an ideal location for conversion into an isolation hospital as part of an initiative driven by the Contagious Diseases Act 1867. This conversion was part of an attempt across England to contain the spread of venereal diseases in Army towns such as Colchester. The plan aimed to administer compulsory treatment to infected prostitutes. The isolation unit started out as a cluster of small, four bedded wards with the addition of temporary structures for periods of high demand. Years later with the onset of smallpox a further twenty bed extension was added and over the years it became the smallpox centre for the north of Essex. After 1910 more blocks needed to be added to treat the First World War troops.

The building and site, taken over by the newly formed National Health Service (NHS) in 1948, was renamed Myland Hospital. As the need for infectious diseases beds reduced, the smallpox ward underwent conversion into a ward for ophthalmic patients and the other wards took general medical and surgical cases. In 1952 a rise in tuberculous patients called for another increase in beds, but within two years the demand decreased again and these beds were reallocated to chronically sick adults who needed respite care. In the 1970s Myland Hospital had one hundred and eighty-one beds, including a geriatric ward. I worked at Myland Hospital in late 1984 and downsize planning had started as the building of the new Colchester General Hospital in nearby Turner Road neared completion. By 1988, with only seventy-seven ophthalmic, geriatric, young chronically sick, and infectious diseases beds open and staffed, the end of its functioning years approached. It finally closed and was demolished in 1989. Whilst working there I often walked through the grounds to the various wards and storage areas, and the locations of the additional wards over the years could easily be spotted. The variety of building materials and their erection style, which included wood, corrugated iron and brick, were a clear give away. The architecture was the only thing I loved about Myland Hospital. The working conditions there formed a depressing and subdued workplace. We often worked with below the recommended staffing levels, meaning that student nurses and auxiliaries picked up the slack. This caused anger and frustration for the doctors and medical professionals who needed experienced staff to support them. As students we wanted to learn, but it was hard with insufficient qualified staff to mentor us. That said, although I

Ooh Matron!

didn't enjoy it I did consider myself fortunate to work with a couple of senior enrolled nurses who took me under their wings. Without them I would not have completed my nurse training. One of them called Pam caught me applying for an office job at a local double glazing factory. She was a large woman with the biggest bust I had ever seen. She put her arms, which appeared short due to her oversized chest, around me in a big motherly maternal hug.

"We need to put a stop to this nonsense Sarah." she said, amongst other things, and from then on things seem to get better. I am not sure if anything really changed or whether she gave me the psychological boost of having a mother figure looking out for me. In the meantime I had got as far as going for an interview at the factory, but luckily they rejected me and suggested I stick to nursing. It turned out to be a lucky escape because my whole life would have been so different if I had not qualified as a nurse.

Before heading into my next hospital-based placement, I was allocated a secondment to the district nursing team to experience their role find and out first-hand how this service links in with pre and post hospital admission care plans. Imagine my surprise and initial horror when the team I became allocated to was not the Colchester based team of district nurses, but the Dovercourt and Harwich team.

Harwich is twenty miles from Colchester and had been home to an international working port since the late 1800s, operating freight and passenger ferries. Harwich developed a salubrious past in the 1970s and 80s when the local Warner's Holiday Camp was used as a filming location for the popular television comedy series 'Hi De Hi!' which starred Sue Pollard. The show, about life in a fictional holiday camp called Maplins after its owner Joe Maplin, was set in a fictional seaside town called Crimpton-on-Sea, Essex. The storylines mimicked the then successful holiday camp company called Butlin's, owned by Billy Butlin.

At the time of this placement I still lived in the hospital house in Colchester and so was offered accommodation at the Dovercourt Cottage Hospital for the days when I would be working there. When I say accommodation I use that term very loosely. This offer was obviously not one taken up very often by student nurses, because the place allocated to me looked uninviting and resembled a temporary storage shed. It was dark, and the metal framed single bed looked like it had come from a ward that Florence Nightingale would have worked on. From the moment I arrived I did not want to stay there, but for the meantime at least I had no choice. There was no opportunity to telephone anyone to try and arrange something else or organise daily transport in line with the shift times.

The district nursing team was small but very friendly, and the first thing I noticed, which they seemed to accept, was that they had far too many patients scheduled in each day to attend within the times allocated. The morning round had to start before 7am to be able to visit all the diabetic patients who needed their insulin injections before breakfast and who were unable to administer it themselves or had no family members to assist them. Some visits which were time-crucial were marked in bold in the diary. This well-used A5 sized diary, with its pages curling up and with some folded over at the corners as reminders looked disorganised, but was used with precision. It contained numerous scraps of paper with telephone numbers, names, addresses, internal memos, etc. stuffed in the back. The first time I was asked to write in it I made sure to write very small, as each page previously was crammed with written notes, appointments, etc. I didn't want to take up too much space on the page.

We would set out at 7am and had four insulin injection visits to make. Some of these patients we would see again later in the day. Then there were personal care visits for bathing or get ups and there were wound care visits, I loved the post-operative surgical wound care because I was familiar with that but there were oh so many leg ulcers being dressed once a week. Harwich and Dovercourt, like many areas on the Essex coast line, were highly populated with retired older people. Often our patients lived in houses that would now not be considered fit for purpose, with their owners suffering from mobility and physical deterioration which compromised their ability to be independent. Many of the houses had been built in the Victorian era and when I saw the first one a tidemark on the side like dirty bath ring, I had to find out how that appeared.

Ooh Matron!

The story goes that during the night of 31 January 1953 the unfortunate combination of a severe storm with a spring high tide resulted in a tidal surge. Property was devastated along the east coast and one hundred and twenty people were killed in Essex. In Harwich a two metre high wave rolled through the main street and eight people drowned. The houses of elderly residents who survived and remained in Harwich wore the tide marks like a symbol of respect. Many of the elderly patients we visited delighted in recounting the tale to a new face visiting.

One of the worst tasks I encountered on this placement was the various bowel treatments we were required to undertake. Many of these measures are no longer in use as clinical evidence now dictates that the risk of internal damage was too high and advancements in medicinal treatments has made these antiquated methods redundant. But at that time it was common place on our rounds to be inserting rectal tubes to assist bedridden constipated patients pass their faeces or stools. The administering of enemas and suppositories every 3rd day, or worse still performing a weekly manual evacuation with only gloves for protection, all fell into my remit as a student. I had never performed a manual evacuation until now. Neither had I inserted rectal tubes, although during my time on Ashley ward I had regularly given suppositories or an enema as preparation for patients needing bowel surgery.

Once I had been shown these two procedures, and demonstrated my ability to perform them they became my responsibility. What do I remember of this new responsibility that I was given? Firstly the smell: it was horrendous and made worse by being in someone's bedroom, surrounded by their personal belongings whilst performing such an invasive, highly embarrassing procedure. This was extremely difficult for a young student nurse to get used to. Secondly, the noise when you insert the rectal tube and the gas exits fast and loud, causing embarrassment for me and the patient. Where do you look? What do you say? Then worse still when the tube is removed what follows is unreal. The first time I removed a rectal tube I thought I had pulled the lining of the patient's large intestine out with the tube. I had to manoeuvre the longest piece of formed stool (poo) I had ever seen into a curly shape to keep it from leaving the bed!

Fortunately there were other more nurse-like tasks that I was given responsibility for during this placement, otherwise I am not sure that I would have made it through. I enjoyed taking down the post-operative dressings from patients discharged after routine operations, and I loved the feeling of satisfaction after removing sutures or clips and being able to observe and record that the wound was 'clean and dry, healing well no signs of infection.'

The scariest set of clips I removed in the community setting was from a woman who had a hysterectomy, (the removal of her uterus or womb as most women refer to it), to treat her fibroids. These are tumours which form and grow in the womb, causing excessive bleeding and painful periods. She was a large woman and even when laying on the bed on her back it took two of us to manipulate her skin folds to expose the wound we needed to remove the clips from, which was on her bikini line. However, I suspected that she had not worn a bikini in many years as it would have got lost. With Sally the district nurse holding the skin away from the wound, I set out my dressing pack and clip remover. As discussed and agreed beforehand, because of the risk of the wound re-opening due to the pressure from the surrounding skin, we were going to remove alternate clips today and then remove the remaining clips 48 hours later. The first two clips came out with no problems; all looked healthy and healing well. However when the third clip released from the skin as I squeezed the slip removers in the palm of my hand, the whole wound started to open. I froze for a second before grabbing a dressing pad and placing it on the wound, holding it firmly over the exposed fatty tissue. Sally calmly said, 'Pop another pack in there Sarah.' Sally carefully lowered the skin fold down covering the packs I had applied and she indicated that we needed to swap sides and roles. I was now on skin holding duty and she would expose the wound and assess the next action that was needed. After a closer examination Sally very gently said to our patient, "I'm really sorry love, but the wound is not healing as we had hoped and I think it would be best if we got you back to the hospital for the surgical team to take a look. It's nothing to worry about."

'Nothing to worry about!' I would be horrified if my abdominal tissue was exposed like that, but thankfully the patient was in unable to see it from any angle. We later found out that the patient had to return to theatre and have her wound re-sutured, no clips this time, and when we returned to remove them all went well.

As my time working in the community drew to an end, I had developed a deep admiration for the work of the district nursing team who, in all weathers and often in unpaid time, worked tirelessly to ensure a high standard of care was provided to their patients. The sense of community in this Essex town and the surrounding areas which we visited was definitely enhanced by the local cottage hospital and the district nurses who helped many people remain in their own homes with family and friends around them. I became an avid fan of the television series 'The District Nurse' which starred Nerys Hughes as nurse Megan Roberts. Although set in a Welsh mining town in 1920s the ethos and community setting in the series was not dissimilar, in many ways, to Harwich and Dovercourt.

It was time to move on professionally and personally, as other changes started to occur during my second year. In my personal life, my mum's health was deteriorating, and I felt guilty pursuing a career and living away from home. At the same time my relationship with Keith struggled, not just because of the travelling distance, but due to the pressures caused by me living in the house share with a reputation for being a haven for party animals. We decided that the answer was to get our own place and move in together. Within a few months we had bought a house in the 1980s property boom in a village on the outskirts of Colchester called Wivenhoe. A small one bedroom Barratt's starter home. The time had come to move out and move on to a new episode in my life and before long we planned to get married.

We married in March 1985 in Stowmarket, Suffolk at the registry office, with a small wedding reception and evening disco in the village hall at Stonham Aspal, the village where I had lived and attended primary school as a child, and where we became regulars at the pub, The Ten Bells, when I stayed at Keith's house on my rest days and holidays. None of my student nurse friends attended, just family and our friends from my life outside of my career.

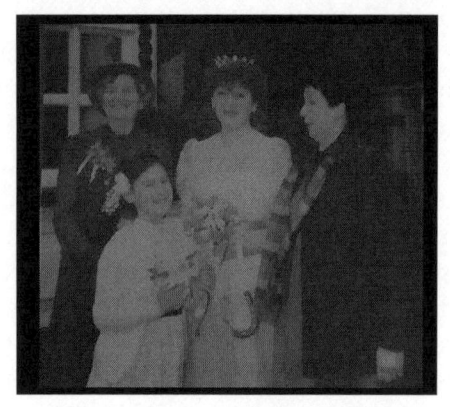

In this photograph from left to right:

Mother of the groom, Dorothy; Sharon, Keith's niece, me and my mum.

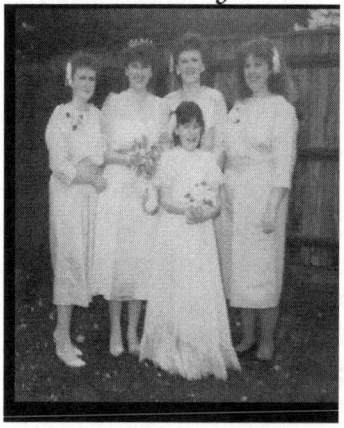

Bridesmaids -Me and my sisters from left to right: Sally, Me, Susie, Evelyn and Sharon at the front.

After a week off it was back to my studies. I had an essay about my district nurse experience that needed to be finished and submitted before I started to prepare for my next speciality placements: gynaecology and obstetrics.

Chapter eight:
Highs and lows of womanhood revealed

As a nineteen year old second year student nurse I gained my first experiences in the world of gynaecology medicine, surgery and obstetrics, better known as maternity care. In the nursing world this is abbreviated to Obs & Gynae. As a woman, although looking back I was still a little immature, my personal experience in this field equalled nil. I had no children and no history of gynaecological problems, therefore the only part familiar to me was the anatomy and physiology of the menstrual cycle, all of which I learned in my human biology O level course. The mere fact that I had moved into female only wards and departments required a very different approach to my work when compared with working in mixed wards and clinics. One of the nicer aspects was that, being a specialism, the conditions, care and treatments were totally focused on specific pieces of anatomy. This was in comparison to the general wards, which carried a wide variety of ages, conditions and outcomes, demanding a wider basic knowledge and skill base for student nurses. Essex County Hospital was the venue for my gynaecological ward placement, which formed part of my 760 hours of surgical placements within my three years training. I worked there for eight weeks on early, late and night shifts.

The age range of the women on the ward during my placement was sixteen to sixty-seven. The range of issues dealt with covered both medical and surgical conditions. Some examples of routine planned surgeries were for conditions such as fibroids which required a hysterectomy and induced abortions. In addition there were emergency surgeries for D& C's or ERPOC after spontaneous abortion or miscarriage, as it is commonly known.

Hysterectomy is the removal of the womb. Sometimes the ovaries are removed as well, which is called an oophorectomy. Removal of the ovaries is dependent on the age of the woman and the condition of the ovaries. I love the word oophorectomy, even though this will sound childish, but because it reminds me of my French language classes at school learning the French word for egg; oeuf.

D& C is dilatation and curettage, or ERPOC (Evacuation of Retained Products of Conception) performed after a miscarriage. This involved having the contents of the womb scraped away to remove any possible tissue fragments or clots which could cause infection.

One particular case that sticks in my mind from my gynaecological placement involved a young couple in their late twenties who had been trying to conceive a baby for about five years. Finally she had a positive pregnancy test and they were taking the first steps towards becoming parents. She was ten weeks pregnant and had been admitted with extreme morning sickness, thought to have been Hyperemesis Gravidarum (excessive nausea and vomiting) and slight vaginal blood spotting, which is not always a problem in pregnancy. It was decided to perform an ultrasound scan (USS) to check that the foetus was growing normally and as a student I was offered the opportunity, with the patients consent, to go and watch the scan. I had never seen this before so I was excited to see a baby in utero and listen to the sonographer explaining everything. I wheeled the patient to the X-ray department after she had drunk a jug of water as she needed a full bladder to help the ultrasound echoes to reach her womb, enhancing the image for the sonographer.

As the patient lay on the couch in the slightly darkened room, with her husband holding her hand, they were still smiling despite her feeling sick and their concern about the spotting. The sonographer applied the lubricating gel, which is put onto the patient's skin to allow the transducer to move smoothly, and ensures that there is continuous contact between the transducer and the skin. Then, the scan probe was moved over the area above her womb. Initially, the screen had been positioned centrally, so that everyone present had a viewpoint, but now the sonographer, with his left hand, started to move the screen towards him instead. I stood behind him, so I still had clear view of the screen. To my inexperienced eyes, not knowing exactly what to look for at such an early stage of pregnancy, confusion reigned at the image that appeared on the screen. It didn't resemble the text book foetus presentation. He asked me to go and ask the registrar to join them which immediately caused anxiety to the young couple. As we waited for the registrar, the time seemed to pass slowly as the sonographer tried to delay and say that he always preferred to consult with the gynaecological surgeon before passing comment on a scan's findings. This did little to reassure them or me.

The registrar walked in and went straight to the screen, some muffled whispering ensued and I reached across and held the woman's free hand, trying to offer something in the way of comfort. The sonographer moved the screen back towards the patient and her husband. He started to point and explain that she had a condition called a Hydatidiform Mole. What the hell! I thought I would be sick at the thought of a black velvety skinned mole burrowing away in her womb. I tried to retain my composure and take in the explanation that it was a condition where the placenta and foetus do not form properly, caused by an imbalance in the chromosomes. Two reasons that this occurs are firstly, if an egg that contains no genetic information is fertilised by a sperm, or secondly a normal egg is fertilised by two sperm. Silence prevailed for what seemed like hours but in reality only minutes. The registrar said he would see the patient back on the ward with the consultant shortly to discuss the treatment. I can't remember the exact words he used to say, 'You're not having a baby' but the pain and despair that consumed them instantly made me cry for the first time in front of a patient. I had been in situations before where I had managed to remove myself from a patient's or visitor's eyeline to let my tears fall, but this was so sudden and unexpected.

The treatment for her Hydatidiform Mole required the surgeon to perform a D&C and send a tissue sample of the 'mole' for examination and histology to try to establish the cause and to check for cancerous cells. Her surgery was booked for that evening at the end of that day's theatre list, so that she could be nil by mouth for four hours, even though she had been sick and it was extremely unlikely that her stomach had any contents left. I saw her the following day on my early shift and she appeared remarkably composed. I can't imagine that I would have been that way. They had been trying for so long to have a baby to then have their dream so crudely snatched away by a genetic abnormality. I hope they did go on to have a child.

My next placement was at the Colchester Maternity Hospital in Lexden Road, Colchester, which opened in 1932 and has since closed in 1997. I delivered all four of my children in this hospital between 1987 and 1996 which was great because some of the older staff I recognised or knew from my training placement. It is a great, imposing building, and despite its age and some of the restrictions resulting from its construction it always felt homely and safe. It is now a development of plush apartments, but its history will remain a big part of Colchester for a many years to come. As a student nurse the schedule of work place experiences that you needed to achieve at the maternity hospital was intensive. I completed 260 hours of practical work during this placement and worked in all areas including ante natal wards and clinics, post-natal wards, the labour suite and home visits with the community midwives and health visitors.

It was always busy and, because of the Colchester garrison, there were sometimes mums without their soldier dads present because their babies decided to arrive early or the dads were away on a tour of duty somewhere. The level of care and support needed varied for each mum and baby and the professionalism of the midwives who mentored and assisted me was exemplary. Many had worked there for years since qualifying, such was the camaraderie and high staff morale there, unlike some of the other wards and hospitals. I loved working in the labour suite and I would have loved to have completed my midwifery training on a post graduate 18 month course when I qualified, but life and relationships got in the way.

Because of the high turnover there was never a shortage of births to witness, this meant that some birthing situations that might normally be rare for a student nurse to observe or be involved in were more accessible. These included emergency caesarean sections, premature births, watching the delivery of a Down's syndrome baby and many more.

I loved the way that each dad coped or dealt with his wife's, girlfriend's or partner's hospital births. Some stayed composed, almost reserved or guarded, as if they feared showing emotion in front of strangers; others revelled in the enormity of the occasion by taking camcorder footage and keeping the whole family in touch with the progress minute by minute. Then there were the single mums who were usually accompanied by their mums or best friends. I found it really hard to see these young girls, some under sixteen and some of whom were totally unprepared for the enormity of the task ahead of them and the huge responsibility that would be theirs after the birth. At the time I had no children of my own and I couldn't imagine what I would have done or how I would have dealt with pregnancy at that age. I love people watching, I am nosey by nature, but working in the delivery suite gave me an opportunity to people watch in unusual circumstances. Without knowing anything of their lives outside of the unit suddenly I could watch and become involved in one of the most important moments of their lives.

There was one particular couple who intrigued me. If you saw them together walking down the street you wouldn't necessarily have thought that they were a couple. She was a tall blonde woman, immaculate makeup, designer label clothes and accessories. He looked like he had been to a pub lock-in for a weekend. He wore creased jeans and a dirty football support shirt, Liverpool or Manchester United, it was red anyway. They were admitted straight to the labour suite as she was already having contractions 3-4 minutes apart when they arrived. On examination her cervix was already 8 cm dilated so for a first baby things were progressing quite fast. After being shown to their room they were asked if they needed any help to get her into a nighty or gown. She took one look at the gown and said words to the effect of 'no way in hell am I wearing that.' However the nighty her husband produced from the bag had obviously been purchased early in the pregnancy when they prepared the hospital bag and to coin her phrase 'there's no way in hell she's going to fit into that;' The midwife Sandra explained that it was the hospital gown or just a sheet as there was no time for another nightdress to be sourced. She went with the sheet, I couldn't believe it, as if childbirth isn't exposing enough. After she clambered in a most un-lady like manner onto the bed, wrapped in a sheet, she then had to manoeuvre herself to become unwrapped from the sheet to enable the midwife to strap her to the foetal heart monitor. At this point she requested the gown and the whole dressing and undressing process started again. Time ticked on and her contractions became more frequent and her swearing increased. Her husband didn't look shocked so perhaps bad language was normal for her. Once she was in the gown and the baby's heart rate had been checked on the monitor, the doctor came in and, after checking the records and talking to Sandra, he said, "Not long now".

"When do I get the epidural?" she said.

"Oh it's too late for that," said Sandra.

The look on the woman's face was one of fear and anger. She accepted the gas and air mask as they debated further analgesia. I made small talk with the husband while Sandra supported his wife. He made a joke about how it was pretty amazing that they managed to get pregnant. Especially as she apparently takes an hour in the bathroom to get ready for bed while he watches television and often falls asleep waiting for her.

Now, picture the scene: football-mad husband at the head end constantly checking his watch like he has bus to catch. Wife in labour vowing that he will never touch her again. Sandra gives her the go-ahead to start pushing on the next contraction.

He is shouting, "Come on! Come on!" as if he's at a football match. He suddenly releases her hand and heads towards the business end of the bed.

"Don't go there you idiot, you'll end up on the floor," she shouts.

He looks a bit insulted at the inference she's made and he stands his ground, just as she starts to push again.

I looked up at his face and tears were falling down his cheeks as he watched the baby's head emerge. He looked up at his wife and said "It's got a head!" Sandra let a smirk develop into a big grin as his wife rolled her eyes in what appeared to be disbelief at his ridiculous comment or his naivety. I wondered what he would say next. I had heard of expectant mums developing baby brain, so perhaps this represented his expectant father baby brain taking over from his normally sensible thought processes. However, he hadn't

Ooh Matron!

presented as the sharpest knife in the drawer since he arrived, so on balance this was probably normal for him.

"Get over here you idiot," she shouted.

I'd never heard a married couple address each other in that way, but it was comical to watch. A healthy baby boy was born which delighted him as he announced, "If they all come out this easily we could form our own footie team". I can't write here what she said next, but I would hazard a guess that you can probably imagine.

Chapter nine:
Mind Matters

The decision to become a nurse, although a last-minute one at age sixteen, did not mean that I doubted in any way that general 'normal' nursing would be my goal. I had no interest in any involvement with psychiatry or areas related to mental health. I am not entirely sure where this deep rooted aversion to these specialties evolved, but the intensity increased after I started my general nurse training. The act of having to walk every day through the grounds of Severalls Hospital from the Mill Road entrance did nothing except reinforce my decision. Severalls Hospital was built in 1910 as one of the original asylums, constructed in Queen Anne style. You can read more on the history of this hospital and its estate in a bonus chapter at the end of this book.

By 1983, and no longer an asylum, only part of the Severalls Hospital still operated psychiatric care beds. It housed three general wards and a few clinics and allied health services, such as occupational therapy, speech therapy and physiotherapy. With general student nurses regularly allocated to the three general wards, I would work on two of them during my three years training. Ashley: the general surgical ward and Jenner: the respiratory medicine ward. However, the psycho-geriatric wards there made my imagination run wild every time I walked through those echoing long corridors. I would hear moaning and crying from old sounding voices when no one could be seen. Was it ghosts of mistreated asylum inhabitants of years gone by, from a time when 'normal' people were locked away for reasons which society now deem 'normal'? Behaviour or accepted conditions and illnesses, such as pregnancy before the age of sixteen and post-natal depression were common reasons for institutionalising women. In some areas of the hospital and in the gardens I would see what I believed to be patients, wandering aimlessly, some sporting the drug induced mask of vacant expression, looking lost and lonely. There were others who were like jovial grandparents and would rush up to you, grab your hands in their hands and tell you how much they missed you. The first time this happened to me I opened my mouth to scream just as a male psychiatric nurse who had been walking behind me in the corridor rushed ahead of me, introduced himself quickly and placed his hands on the old man's shoulders.

"Joe you startled the young lady, now let's introduce ourselves properly as you will probably be seeing a fair bit of each other."

Gavin, the male nurse, obviously recognised the tell-tale signs of a new student nurse and probably carried out this rescue mission frequently.

By my second year, as the time approached for my eight week placement in psychiatry and mental health, I had not grown any fonder of the speciality even though I had become used to meeting the psycho-geriatric patients in the corridors. I knew this would be one of the hardest placements during my three years in training. My allocation was a split placement with a secure unit in East Hill near the Castle Park in Colchester town centre, which accommodated 'residents', not patients, with a variety of mental health issues and disabilities. However, the majority were Down's syndrome young adults aged eighteen to thirty-five during my time there. This placement was an enlightening and, as it turned out, humbling experience for me. Although I knew a few people in our local area with Down's syndrome children, having never given any thought to them and therefore with no understanding of the issues faced as they reached adulthood, I remained in blissful ignorance. The issues around coping with adulthood and their personal health increased if they had been born to older parents. Medical evidence at that time indicated that pregnancy in women over the age of thirty-five increased the risk of conceiving a Down's syndrome baby. Therefore with less information for prospective parents, limited screening or prenatal testing, the incidence increased in the thirty-five to forty-five years age range. One of the problems this created was that by the time these children reached adulthood, their parents would be approaching their late fifties or sixties and might possibly have health issues of their own to deal with.

Sarah Jane Butfield

Some of the health issues Down's syndrome children and young adults can present with and which require additional medical management in adulthood include:

- Thyroid imbalances and diabetes
- Depression and obsessive-compulsive disorder (OCD)
- Musculoskeletal issues and spinal cord compression
- Periodontal disease, cataracts and hearing loss or impairment
- Epilepsy and sleep apnoea
- Heart valve disease
- Skin problems and eczema.

One of the other more fundamental issues to be accommodated in a mental health unit housing male and female residents was sex! With all residents having reached puberty, normal adult behaviours and desires existed in their minds and bodies. Although males with Down's syndrome predominantly have a lower rate of fertility, as a preventative measure the females, whenever possible and with family consent, were prescribed the contraceptive pill. At that time the contraceptive injection, depot medroxyprogesterone acetate, which was marketed as Depo-Provera, started to become more widely used, but the contraceptive pill remained commonplace. However, there was little to be done to halt the desire for intimacy and it would be a regular occurrence to find them canoodling, in various stages of undress, in cupboards and bedrooms if left unattended for any length of time.

No more than two student nurses worked in the unit at any one time so you never worked on the same shift as another student, and we were not permitted to work nights. We would take part in providing supervision with personal care as they were encouraged to maintain as much independence as possible and the other role was to escort them to social and therapeutic appointments. This involved taking them to the local pub, The Foresters Arms in Castle Road, two evenings a week, visiting the cafe in Castle Park and going on a variety of shopping trips. Contrary to my initial reservations I actually enjoyed this placement. I learned a great deal about coping with the stigma of society in relation to mental

disability, which wears a prominent mask in the form of the visual recognition of Down's syndrome adults.
- The most obvious and easily recognisable are the slanting eyes, small external ears and large tongues in comparison to their small mouths.
- A flattened bridge of the nose, which is more obvious on their characteristically small nose.
- Short fingers on hands with a small width can reduce dexterity.
- Down's syndrome sufferers tend to be shorter in height than an adult of similar age, with shorter necks which makes their facial features appear more prominent. In babies and young children the characteristics are easy to see but often induce a loveable sympathetic reaction. In adulthood these physical features leave them open to discrimination and abuse.

On shopping trips I immediately became defensive, especially when groups of teenagers would shout abuse at them or make jokes about them. Our instructions were not to interact if such behaviour took place, but you have to bear in mind that some of the residents demonstrated some immature characteristics which provoked these outbursts and made dealing with them all the more taxing. That said, they could on occasion put these perpetrators in their place with one of their party tricks, such as pretending to have a seizure, which was a favourite of Eddie, one of the oldest residents who I enjoyed spending time with. Eddie was about forty-seven, which at that time for a Down's syndrome male was considered quite old, due to the complexity of physical health issues that they usually faced. In coffee shops or restaurants if he wanted to get served, as waitresses tended to ignore us, probably in the hope we would get fed up with waiting and go somewhere else. Eddie wore glasses and, if he wanted to get served, he would take his glasses off and wave them in the air and start singing Tom Jones, 'Green, Green Grass of Home.' Nobody wanted his singing in their establishment so they served him quickly to keep his mouth occupied.

Sarah Jane Butfield

The feigning of seizures, a trick that he taught some of the younger residents as a way to make abusive teenagers leave them alone, caught me out a few times until another staff member filled me in on the background to this behaviour. The strategy for using this included firstly giving a sign to the member of staff accompanying them so they knew it was fake. The signs, either patting the top of their heads or saying 'I really need to poo now!' proved quite ambiguous at busy times in the town centre. As a student I never went out alone with a resident we always went in a group of four to six with one or two of the regular staff in attendance. The first time I saw the fake seizure routine I had not been made privy to the 'signs' so it alarmed me that the staff members with me did not intervene when a potential seizure started. However, I soon got used to it.

One of the most endearing Down's syndrome characteristics is that on the whole they can be loving and openly display uninhibited signs of affection. The number of times in a day one or other of the residents would tell me that they loved me and would give me a big hug, could raise a smile even on the hardest days. As the unit, not located within the hospital grounds, was not an acute establishment there were only facilities to deal with basic first aid. This meant that we became regular attendees at the nearby accident and emergency department after falls, fights and kitchen accidents. Cooking or meal preparation with the residents proved hilarious, at times. To maintain independence and teach life skills to facilitate the opportunity for home visits or transfer to a less secure unit with fewer staff we encouraged independence with personal care activities, and also with planning and preparation of snacks and meals. Lunch time often involved sandwich making and, given the opportunity, this ended up in food fights and food combinations that would make you cringe. The fridge always had cheese, ham, butter and various salad items. The pantry was always stocked with tins of soup, canned fish, baked beans and multiple jars of peanut butter, marmite, jams and spreads. The residents who suffered from diabetes or any other dietary affected conditions were allocated their foods to make sandwiches with, but the others helped themselves. Now, as with children, if they saw someone having something different and especially something they had been told

Ooh Matron!

they were not allowed, this often resulted in angry outbursts, food being thrown at the walls or the staff and sometimes deceptive behaviour.

On one occasion as I supervised Mark, one of the diabetics who was making a tuna salad, things turned sour. Mark chopped his spring onions, sliced the cucumber and had just started on the tomatoes as Jean entered the kitchen. Jean, a resident in her late fifties, did not have Down's syndrome, but she presented with a similar mentality and borderline physical characteristics. She worked unsupervised and started preparing to make a toasted sandwich. I had seen her unsupervised in the kitchen before and so I didn't think anything of it. However, on this occasion she plastered both sides of the four slices of white bread with chocolate spread making a sticky mess on the worktop, which was what first attracted both Mark's and my attention.

When she then proceeded to start spreading Marmite on top of the chocolate spread I said, "Jean that may not taste too good, shall we get some more bread and start again?"

Big mistake on my part. She picked up the slices of bread and ran towards me. As she got closer she raised her hand as if to slap my face with the bread slice, when Mark suddenly pounced on her. They both landed on the floor and all went quiet, too quiet for a few seconds. Dee, one of the managers heard the commotion and came running in and together we prised Mark and Jean apart. My initial fear was that Mark still had the knife in his hand from the salad preparation, but luckily it still lay on the work surface. However, he did have a squashed tomato in his left hand and Jean now wore the slices of chocolate spread covered bread on her blouse. Within seconds of getting them to a sitting position we collapsed into fits of hysterical laughter. If anyone had looked in at that moment who knows that they would have thought had happened? Mark suddenly blurted out, "Are you ok Miss Sarah?"

"Yes Mark, thank you."

"Was I your hero?"

I looked at Dee and then back to Mark, "Mark no one has ever protected me like that before so you are definitely my hero."

Dee took Jean through to the bathroom to help her clean up. When they returned Jean apologised for her behaviour like a child told by their parent to apologise to a neighbour for kicking the ball over the fence. She apologised, but did not mean it.

After the kitchen was cleared up and with lunch eaten we made Mark a badge which said 'Miss Sarah's hero' and he wore it for days afterwards. All the male residents called me Miss Sarah, and I really missed that when I moved on to the second part of my psychiatric/mental health placement in which the patients behaved in a more distant self-protecting manner.

The next stop for me would be working with patients who had attempted suicide and were being cared for not only in the hospital environment, but also in the community as I would be accompanying the community psychiatric nurse on home visits. In the dark recesses of my mind I remembered a story talked about in my childhood, concerning an attempted suicide. I don't know for sure, even to this day, if any truth lay within that story. However, in hindsight it's possible that the memory of this story subconsciously influenced my aversion to this placement and the trouble I experienced settling in to it and coming to terms with the reasons, often misunderstood, about why people attempt suicide.

To be honest as I wrote this chapter I struggled to recall any events or experiences that I would feel comfortable to share in this book in relation to my psychiatric placement. Not because they were traumatic or disturbing, but because I genuinely feel that I wasn't either mature or experienced in life enough to appreciate, absorb or understand the rationale behind the varying levels of psychosis and psychiatric conditions that I was exposed to. I did find the link between certain medical conditions and the development of psychosis interesting, such as thyroid disorders, Lupus and Cushing Syndrome. The fact that sleep deprivation can present as psychosis I found quite alarming. Therefore I concluded that I definitely made the right decision to choose general nursing.

Ooh Matron!

Chapter ten:
Theatrical high jinks and honey traps

Since the start of my training, surgery and anything to do with it strongly appealed to me. I think the concept and sense of achieving a tangible result from a defined intervention piqued my interest, whereas medical nursing appeared more probing and investigative, and to my mind involved a more often long winded approach. I was excited knowing that I would have a placement in the operating theatre suite during my training and this meant that I always took a keen interest in the recovery area whenever I went to collect post-operative patients to escort them back to the ward. Regardless of the surgery, the procedure for pre and post-operative delivery and return was standard. A nurse or student would escort the patient to the anaesthetic area, complete the identity and operation confirmation checks and then leave them to undergo their surgery. Later, theatre recovery room staff would call to request the patient be collected from the recovery area when they had come round from the anaesthetic and were stable enough to return to the ward area for continuous monitoring.

By the time my placement date arrived the operating theatre suite had relocated to the new Colchester Hospital; originally named the District General Hospital (DGH) and later re-branded as Colchester General Hospital. (CGH) Since it opened and the transition of the wards and services had started, the Essex County Hospital and the theatres there became specialist areas, and the general wards, theatres and their staff started to transfer to DGH. Working in a brand new hospital in a prestigious, some would say elitist, department gave student nurses and especially me a thrill. We had access to areas of the hospital unavailable to other staff, not for our own use, but to run errands for the medical and nursing teams. It was this elite mentality that gave way to a range of superiority complexes amongst the theatre staff and for this reason, if another department or group of staff found an opportunity to knock them off their pedestals, then they took it in a quick, clean and public arena.

The performance of surgery, whether as a routine planned operation or emergency life saving measure, involves a team approach, and for all the bravado and jealously from other departments the one element of working in this environment which I enjoyed and respected was that they planned, worked and supported each other as a team at all times. Being a smaller team than most areas and being specialised in their individual roles and responsibilities meant that they relied heavily on each member to perform their roles to the highest possible standards. A single error or misjudged action jeopardised the department and had the ability to make this vulnerable house of cards collapse. When students worked in the department the staff were careful to ensure that we would receive a thorough induction to enable us to perform tasks within our range of growing skills and be able to contribute as a valued theatre team member. This, in my experience, had not been the case in some of the specialised departments I worked in to date, where some senior staff would prefer to make you sit and read procedure manuals than to teach hands-on skills which was the expectation on our 'practical' placements.

The operating theatre suite was divided into three main areas, anaesthetics, theatres and recovery. Each area had its own team of staff and lead nurse, however one operating theatre department sister position existed to manage the day to day running in relation to staff, training, support and compliance. In the main, only the surgical team doctors moved between the three areas. The consultant anaesthetist led the pre-operative area and a senior staff nurse led the nursing team. In the actual theatres there were scrub nurses, who prepared and handed all the instruments, equipment and so on to the surgeons and assisted as instructed. In the recovery area the senior staff nurse had a team of staff and enrolled nurses. As student nurses we spent two week in anaesthetics, and three weeks in theatres and the recovery area.

Anaesthetic room activities for student nurses focused on the observation of protocols and procedures in relation to patient safety. This involved the checking, and double checking any element that

Ooh Matron!

might impact on the surgical procedure about to be undertaken or the post-operative period.

- Have we got the right patient, (right name, date of birth, hospital number, have they got two separate name bands, etc.)?
- Is there a signed consent form for the planned operation or procedure?
- Do they have any allergies to medications, sticky tape or even food as some medicines can contain food based ingredients such as egg protein which can cause a reaction?
- Are there any underlying conditions or issues which could be affected by anaesthetic procedures or could cause complications during surgery? If so, are they clearly documented and are the surgical team fully aware of them?

One of the student nurse assigned tasks was less appealing to a young inexperienced woman like me. When male patients were prepared on the ward for a vasectomy or male sterilisation in the 1980s, the procedure dictated that their pubic region be shaved. It was not permissible for them to do it themselves and on the wards student nurses were often allocated this task. Once in my theatre placement I anticipated a temporary reprieve from this task, but I soon realised how many trained staff skipped the shaving when no students were around to allocate it, to thus sending the male patient to theatre unprepared. If the anaesthetic room staff spotted this, they would make the student in anaesthetic area complete the shave. If it happened on a regular basis in the course of a day, the consultant would sometimes instruct the anaesthetic room nurse to return the patient to the ward and reschedule the operation, obviously not a desirable outcome. Fortunately for me, during my two weeks in anaesthetics, I only had to complete it once, unlike some of my fellow students. On the ward, you performed the shave behind the bedside curtains, just you and the patient, which is bad enough. In theatre you are observed by the anaesthetist, ODAs

Sarah Jane Butfield

(Operating Department Assistants) and the anaesthetic room nurses. Imagine picking up the floppy penis of an anxious, usually young man, holding it out of harm's way while you shave around it. This disconcerting task for a student was highly embarrassing for the patient. One man on the ward once said, "Holy shit, if I get a hard on I am so sorry!"

The learning curve spiked from day one. My head ached from trying to remember the checking procedures and the constant quizzing of the anaesthetist. This was his tried and trusted method of ensuring that we developed the knowledge he needed us to have to function in his domain.

Some of the ODAs who assisted in many aspects of theatre life often instigated practical jokes within the department, especially with new staff. After my stint in anaesthetics I excitedly made the move into shadowing the scrub nurses in the theatres. The lighting, the surgeon's choice in music being played and the fear of touching anything that could contaminate this sterile area was overwhelming. You can imagine that, on my first time in theatre, what I did not need was to be the subject of the ODAs' practical jokes. The morning orthopaedic list, which included two knee replacements, a below knee amputation and some pin and plate procedures, got underway. I had nursed patients during the post-operative period of leg amputations on Ashley Ward, so I was really interested in the amputation procedure to try to piece together how what happens in theatre can implicate the post-operative period. I obviously made my interest in the amputation too obvious because it provided the ODAs with all the material they needed to target me.

Imagine the scene. We are in the operating theatre, the patient is laying on the operating table anaesthetised. The surgeons are scrubbing in and the scrub nurses are already in position. As there was a limb removal scheduled there were two ODAs in the theatre instead of one. My allocated position, designed to keep me out of the way, was near the wall beside a large bin lined with a yellow bag. I had watched the two knee replacements that morning and so I was confident that there was nothing about the amputation procedure that would make feel unwell or faint. The sin of all sins for student nurses. The operation got underway and the leg which had been marked with a black arrow was covered in drapes exposing just the incision site. The surgeon started making the skin incision and called for the diathermy, to cauterise the blood vessels. Then he requested the saw to cut through the bone. At this point the ODAs moved in towards the operating table. Due to their presence, my view became obscured but I could hear what was happening with the saw and the suction machine.

Then David one of the ODAs shouted, "Bring us the bucket girl." He looked straight at me. With no one behind me it was obvious his request was intended for me. I reached down, grabbed the bucket and took a step towards the table.

My approach was suddenly interrupted as the other ODA, Mark, shouted, "Catch!" Something, hurtled towards me and the bucket. I lifted it up just as the object, which looked like a limb, landed in the bucket. However, it landed with such force that I dropped the bucket under the sudden weighted pressure as it forced the release of my feeble grip from the shiny plastic lining of the bucket. Everyone looked at me.

I looked across to Mark who had thrown the object just as David shouted, "Holy crap it's the wrong leg." With everyone still looking at me, I could feel my eyes welling up with tears, but I did not really know why. After all, I hadn't cut the wrong leg off! Then as I stood there, not daring to look down at the bucket in case the leg had found its way out and onto the floor, which would have been mortifying, hysterical laughter broke out. Mark stepped towards me and picked up the bucket, lifting out not the amputate limb but a prosthetic leg. By now I was shaking as the laughter continued. After they regained their composure, and I took a few deep breaths, the operation continued and the surgeon asked me to join the scrub nurse at the table.

After the operation David led me into the scrub room and said, "Sorry luv, that was funny, at least you didn't pass out or run away. Bloody good catch! I think you'll fit in just fine here."

The next time I saw a trick played in theatre, it was on a trainee ODA and they were much harsher with him.

Theatres in the DGH were manned 24/7, and overnight the doctors on duty had use of the on-call rooms, in the hope they would get some rest or sometimes even sleep in between being paged to attend the wards or attend emergencies. As students in a speciality department, we were not on the rota for night duty because of inadequate numbers of supervisory staff to support us. However, at the end of a late shift, staff of all grades would often hang out in the theatre staff tea room or sometimes congregate in one of the on-call rooms to plan meet ups at the pub or at one of the doctor's houses in Turner Road opposite the hospital. Just like any large establishment where male and female staff work together, workplace romances and relationships can and do develop. With shift work and a home and family life thrust into the equation, the juggling act to keep all of those balls in the air was tough. Some staff however not only managed that, but also made time for additional relationships in the form of work place affairs.

In theatres there was one particular member of staff who was a prolific flirt, we will call him Brian. He targeted any new female staff regardless of their job, grade or qualifications. Domestic staff, students, qualified nurses or junior doctors, no female was exempt. Despite his reputation being widely known and regularly a topic of discussion in both the theatre staff room and the main hospital canteen, still women fell for it. He was nothing great to look at either, but he had the 'gift of the gab' as they say in Essex. He could charm the birds from the trees. To give you an idea of his looks, have you seen the film 'True Lies' starring Arnold Schwarzenegger and Jamie Lee Curtis? No he was not an Arnie look-alike, he was the mousey moustached, car sales guy Simon, played by Bill Paxton, both in his looks and mannerisms. In the film, Simon pretends to be a spy to seduce vulnerable bored housewives. Well that's what Brian looked and acted like. One weekend the theatres were quiet, no emergencies and we were doing the 'weekend cleaning', special jobs designed to keep all grades of nursing and operating theatre staff occupied in-between emergencies at weekends. Jobs such as cleaning specialised equipment that needed to be dismantled; clearing out cupboards and checking expiry dates on autoclaved instruments, etc. Anyway in our tedium, we started discussing honey traps. The conversation inevitably ended up with the conclusion that it would be fun for Brian to get pay back for his flirty and adulterous behaviour. As the conversation developed so did the idea of catching him out in a honey trap.

Ooh Matron!

The definition of a honey trap is, 'a scheme in which a victim is lured into a compromising sexual situation to provide an opportunity for blackmail'. We had no intention of blackmailing Brian per se, but we did hope to deter him from his flirtatious behaviour. Even though he appeared to show no preference for a particular type of woman we decided that for the best chance we should 'use', or perhaps enlist the help of sounds nicer, someone with the looks required for this exercise: the stereotypical long legged blonde. I knew just the person. Alicia from my class was currently on allocation in the children's ward and not enjoying the experience, so she was game for any excuse to mix with some grown-ups and she was up for getting involved.

So with the willing participant in place we needed to set the trap. Brian didn't wear a wedding ring and never spoke about his wife or children and this fact, combined with his blatant behaviour, inflamed tensions among some of the theatre staff. The plan revolved around enticing Brian to chat up Alicia and invite her to the on-call room, his usual chat up line, where he liked to get to know new staff better. However, not wanting to put Alicia at risk our plan required making sure the on-call room was occupied, to see what he would suggest instead. It all seemed innocent enough in theory and we were only fact-finding about his alternative rendezvous spots. I invited Alicia down to the theatre staff room. Brian would be on duty with Mark who told Brian that Alicia would be coming to find out about risk factors in relation to children during surgery for a project. We added those details as it was possible Brian would have seen her before on the children's ward when collecting or delivering patients from theatre, even though she had only been there two weeks.

On cue Alicia arrived, looking fabulous as ever, and I sat talking to her in the staff room until Brian came in. I was then 'called away' to see a specimen of interest for my project which conveniently left Alicia and Brian alone. Within five minutes, he walked down towards the doors that led to the on-call rooms with Alicia in tow. You had to give this guy marks for consistency and his ability to speed date. The on-call rooms were occupied or so Brian was led to believe by the fact that they were locked. We waited for Brian and

Alicia to double back and find somewhere else to 'chat'. We waited. They didn't come back. We looked at each other; this was not going to plan.

"Someone has to go down there and see where they are?" said Nolene one of the scrub nurses. They all looked at me. "She's your friend you need to go and check on her". No discussion, no debating, decision made by Nolene. I opened the door and walked past the on-call rooms. All doors closed. I didn't try the handles in case they had managed to get inside one of them. Imagine if I tried the door and it opened, what excuse could I have for trying the door of an on-call room? As I neared the end of the passageway I heard muffled talking and giggling. As I turned to walk back towards theatres I heard it again, but louder, coming from the linen store. I opened the door and there they were bold as brass kissing and getting it on. "Give us a minute babe will you?" Brian said.

I quickly turned and shut the door firmly as I left. I hated being called 'Babe' especially by him. As I walked back into theatres Nolene said, "Well, did you find them?"

"Oh yes, I found them alright, some honey trap that turned out to be she's snogging his face off in the linen store!"

The pair of them emerged soon after and Alicia made no apologies for her behaviour. Brian's smug expression irritated everyone and we avoided him for the remainder of the shift. Our plan foiled by a blonde. A few months after this event Alicia found a doctor to cosy up to in a treatment room and guess who found her? Yes, you guessed it, me.

Ooh Matron!

Chapter eleven:
By Royal appointment.

In 1977 as a twelve year old member of the Coddenham Girl Guides in rural Suffolk, it was a memorable royal year for me. First, one of the over sixteen year old Girl Guides in our troupe, Zena, was awarded the prestigious Queen's Guide Award which was the highest award that could be achieved in the Girl Guides. Second, we awaited news of the planned local celebrations for Queen Elizabeth II's Silver Jubilee. A range of special engagements would be taking place around the UK, but for the Girl Guides in Suffolk, as local groups, we discussed and were eager to undertake our roles and get involved in helping to organise and take part in parties, fetes and events to celebrate this royal occasion.

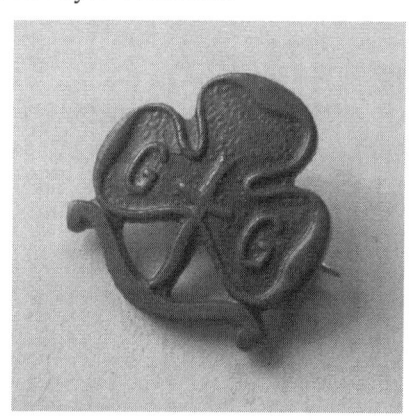

My Girl Guide badge used to secure my cross over uniform tie

However, as part of the official celebrations for the Silver Jubilee, Queen Elizabeth II would tour and visit various hospitals, schools, businesses and church community projects. The scheduled visit on 11th July 1977 to the nearby town of Ipswich would include a visit to the Cornhill in the town centre and St Clement's Hospital in Foxhall Road on the outskirts. These would be the nearest places that the Queen would visit close to where I lived and as I loved to collect newspaper clippings of anything to do with the Royal family I eagerly awaited the coverage by the local newspapers the East Anglian Daily Times and the Ipswich Evening Star. A few selected representatives from the Rangers, Girl Guides, Brownies, Boy Scouts, Cubs, etc., would be invited to line the route for the Queen's visit to the hospital. Therefore, imagine my surprise, excitement and delight when I received the letter informing me I had been chosen as one of the Girl Guide representatives for the South East Suffolk Guide Division. Even though the letter came addressed to 'Coddenham Guide (sorry but I haven't your name)' nothing could detract from the sense of occasion, maybe I would even get my picture in the newspaper. To be selected as part of the representation for this special occasion was a tremendous honour. Not only to be able to see the Queen close up rather than in the newspaper or on television, but to actually be chosen from the hundreds of Girl Guides in the Suffolk area to represent the Girl Guide organisation. This was a huge event in our household and my mum was so proud.

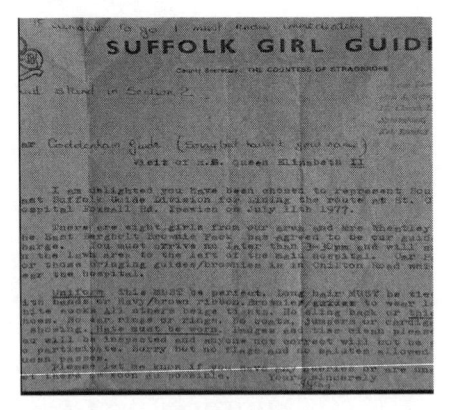

Official letter of invitation

My letter of invitation had clear, detailed instructions on the timings, location of assembly points and uniform etiquette, with the most important aspects typed in capital letters. With no margin for error our Girl Guide leader made sure I had a full uniform trial run before the day and I was given packets of spare tights and hairgrips

Ooh Matron!

to ensure that my tights had no holes or ladders and that whatever the weather my hat stayed in place. The day of the Queens' visit was over far too quickly for me. However, as usual mum collected and kept all the newspaper clippings from the visit by Queen Elizabeth II, even though I didn't appear in any of them, so that we could relive the memories any time we pleased.

Eight years later in the summer of 1985, during my second year placement on the children's ward, I found myself in the right place to be in the presence of the Queen again. This time it was as she visited to officially open the £16 million first phase of the new Colchester General Hospital.

The opportunity to meet or just get a passing glimpse of the Queen as a student nurse was no less exciting or nerve-wracking than when I was a Girl Guide. Those of us that were student and pupil nurses and who would be part in the line-up or possibly within eye shot of the Queen, her party or members of the media at various places within the new Colchester General Hospital along the Queens route were subjected to rigorous coaching and preparation by our tutors in the weeks leading up to the visit. If deemed necessary for whatever reason, such as hems too high, too low or frayed, etc., we were able to go and acquire a brand new uniform dress. New dresses came pressed so full of starch that they could have stood up independently to welcome Queen Elizabeth II. We also had our white belts inspected by Mr Waters, our tutor, and were issued with a brand new white belt if ours showed any signs of stains, which most of ours did as second year students. My well-used belt, which was routinely scrubbed with an old toothbrush, had a definitive grey tinge to it by this time.

Our tutors made the preparations more rigorous than the ward sister, with a checklist of what we should and could not wear or look like; it was extensive. I believe in hindsight, to make their selection and adherence to these strict protocols easier, they deliberately picked students who pretty much adhered to uniform policy in the first place. As you can probably imagine, by this stage of our training, some of my class mates had already changed their regulation black lace up shoes for more fashionable versions, and the levels of make-up and the tidiness of their hair was decreasing

as our time as student nurses ticked on. The line-up was not purely made up of student nurses, there were staff from all departments in the hospital being prepared for the occasion.
For student and pupil nurses the rules of engagement for this honourable occasion were simple and to be strictly enforced:

- No jewellery except a wedding band
- Natural looking or no make-up
- Hair neat if short or tied back and well secured if long
- Black lace up, low heeled shoes, polished
- 40 denier black tights
- Fingernails short neatly trimmed and no nail varnish
- Name badges must be worn on the right and pinned level with the top fastening of the uniform dress
- Clean unmarked white belt secured with Velcro and not safety pins.

The line-up practice and positioning, even for those that would not be the closest to the Queen as she walked from the main front entrance to the children's ward, still had the reinforcement of the rule, 'Do not attempt to speak to the Queen'. What would you say anyway? "Hello, lovely weather isn't it?"

On 17th May 1985, the day before my 20th birthday, Queen Elizabeth II visited Coggeshall Ward, which was the children's ward at that time. On the morning of the visit there was a buzz of excitement on the ward and throughout the hospital as staff of all grades readied themselves and the hospital communal and ward areas that would be visited or passed through. Before her arrival at the Colchester General Hospital the Queen would be visiting the Colchester University and meeting the mayor at the Colchester Town Hall for lunch. At the hospital, security was in place and ancillary staff rolled pieces of red carpet out and vacuumed them countless times so that they would be ready and waiting to be used at the precise pre-planned moments. Photography other than by the media was banned for all staff. The visit passed off uneventfully. Once on the ward the Queen chatted with patients, staff and family members who were visiting their children. I was positioned near to the ward entrance. The Consultant Paediatrician and the Ward

Ooh Matron!

Sister took the Queen on the tour of Coggeshall Ward and I felt very proud just to witness the occasion.

I have to admit that I was anxious and apprehensive about nursing children as a non-parent, at the time, during my placement on the children's ward. I wondered if I would have enough empathy for the parents, as I had limited experience of children who were in good health let alone sick ones, and I prepared myself to be tested by this experience. That said, it was an eye opening experience and the memory of some of the patients and their families have stayed with me throughout my now almost twenty-eight years as parent myself. The tube feeding of tiny babies with feeding problems due premature birth, cardiac or respiratory medical conditions was a skill that evoked much fear initially. The complications and risks associated with incorrect feeding preparation or methods could ultimately result in the feed going into the baby's lungs, therefore the practical training in this procedure, for very good reasons, was intense and well supervised. It was sad, but in a strange way satisfying to become part of the skilled, multi-purpose allied health team that supported and cared for the children suffering from conditions such as Cystic Fibrosis, Coeliac Disease and Congenital Heart Defects, etc. These children and their families were, or became, regular in-patients and visitors. Often, my being a new student on the ward, the children I cared for knew more about their condition and treatment than I did. Some of them could even show me how to use the specialised equipment because they had a similar set up at home. The range and scope of practice needed and utilised within this one area of healthcare was vast. The patients requiring nursing care and treatment of medical conditions like these were nursed alongside children attending for short-stay planned medical, surgical and day case interventions and treatments, such as blood or platelet transfusions, intravenous antibiotic therapy, etc. The planned surgical cases dealt with elective procedures for ear, nose and throat (ENT) conditions including adenoids problems, fitting grommets for glue ear, dental issues dealing with problematic teeth and gums and orthopaedic cases for broken bones or joint related issues. These and many more childhood related conditions kept us on our toes on the routine theatre days. However, when emergency cases presented on top of this, as was normal, then the reality was that the children's ward remained at full occupancy and extremely busy.

The other difference in working in this environment was that the majority of children had a parent or family member who stayed with them throughout their stay, particularly the babies and young children. Some of the children with chronic conditions who regularly had in-patient admissions to the ward didn't always have anyone and so the importance of recognising that they needed entertaining, education and company or attention during their stay was crucial.

One of the hardest elements of working on the children's ward for me was when children were admitted for treatment and investigation of unexplained injuries. In some of these cases the students were allocated the task of having to supervise the parents or close family while they visited or played with their child. Working with the play therapist gave me a great insight into how children deal with traumatic events and how in some cases they subconsciously try to reinvent themselves to prevent further abuse or neglect. The use of toys, games and role play can give a child a medium through which to tell their story without directly implicating the abuser, but giving enough information for health visitors, social workers and sometimes police officers to investigate further. The security of babies and children as inpatients was, and is, of paramount importance and it is good to see, and know, that it has increased over the years since I worked in the maternity units and children's ward. Today, in the majority of maternity and special care baby units across the UK, there is some form of electronic security device in the cots. In some the cot mattresses are alarmed to go off when the baby is lifted out unless the key allocated to the mother, nurse or midwife is inserted to turn off the alarm. This allows the mother to be able to leave her baby temporarily unattended in safety while she visits the toilet, or nurses station for advice, etc. Entrances to children wards and units with vulnerable patients, in the main, are operated by remotely activated locking systems so that visitors have to ring the bell, announce themselves via an intercom and say who they are and who they wish to visit. The staff decide who they let in. For example, if it is an inconvenient time for the patient, a rest period or if someone is already with the child, access may be denied. These measures and many more like them have improved the safety and security of babies and children in hospital.

I am very proud that thirty years after I worked on the children's ward my step daughter Clair has just graduated as a paediatric nurse.

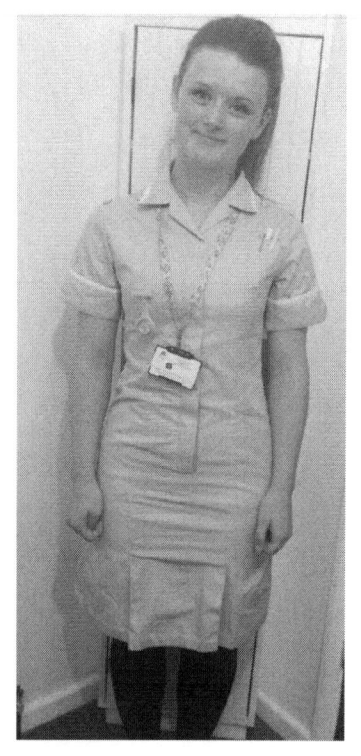

Paediatric Staff Nurse - Clair Victoria Butfield

She studied at the Anglia Ruskin University and worked, among other places, on the new children's unit, built and opened in 2011 within the same hospital in which I trained and worked, the original Colchester General Hospital.

Sarah Jane Butfield

There have been many changes over the last thirty years not least of which means that instead of having Coggeshall children's ward as the only dedicated children's area the children's unit now consists of:

- Children's Assessment Unit with 8 emergency beds for acute cases
- Children's Elective Care Unit with 10 beds for planned admissions for day case care and surgery
- Children's Inpatient Ward with 24 beds including 2 high dependency beds
- Children's outpatient department, a huge bonus as it is completely dedicated to children.

Chapter twelve:
Student nurse training now

Although there are many elements of student nurse training's delivery, assessment and examination which have changed over the last thirty years, some aspects and in particular the personal psychological experiences are similar. I have asked Clair, my step-daughter, who has just completed her three years of paediatric nurse training at The Anglia Ruskin University and Colchester Hospitals, to write a short piece to help demonstrate the similarities and differences, then versus now. It has been great to be able to share her student nurse journey whilst remembering and documenting my own.

Welcome Clair.

Student nurse training 1983- 1986 versus 2012 – 2015 by Clair Victoria Butfield

Thank you so much for asking me to contribute to your book, I am a bit nervous about it but here we go.

It's July 2015 and I am sitting in the sun on my day off from placement, looking back on the past three years of my nurse training, smiling at the thought that in just two months' time I will be wearing a hat and gown, celebrating my graduation and qualifying as a paediatric nurse. To say the last three years has been an incredible experience would somewhat be an understatement; it has been an emotional roller coaster. I have endured some of my worst days, but certainly not forgetting I have also experienced my best.

Looking back to September 2012, my first weeks at Anglia Ruskin University in Chelmsford, Essex, I received an overload of vital information. I can't speak for how nurse training commenced when Sarah was first starting, but now you spend three or four months in university for theory sessions and lectures before being exposed to the clinical environment of the hospital or community setting, piling on information about the anatomy and physiology of the infant, child and young person, common conditions, basic assessment of an unwell child... to name a few. As well as this, we also had three exams to prepare for on professional issues in nursing, anatomy and physiology and medication administration, which we undertook in December 2012, before our break for Christmas. A lot of information and skills training is squeezed into the first few months of nursing training, and in the beginning all you want to do is get into the hospital and start being a nurse. But looking back, we all needed that time to build up our knowledge and skills before being exposed to the real nursing environment. The university has fantastic facilities for practicing basic nursing skills such as taking a blood pressure, administering medications and dressing a variety of wounds, all of which we, as students, were given the opportunity to master before we started our first nursing placements in January 2013.

Even now, three years on, my first day of a new placement is terrifying, but nothing in comparison to how I was feeling on my first day on my first ever placement on the Children's Elective Care Unit. My first ever 7am start was a challenge in itself (now something that has become a normality in my life), not to mention trying to remember where everything was during my orientation, the routine of the day and who everyone was. I was assigned my mentor, a fantastic nurse who I will always remember, and began to shadow her during everything she did. At first I felt a little like a lost sheep, my mentor was so knowledgeable and such a natural nurse. I almost felt as though I would never be able to get to that stage and be so confident and competent in what I did. I think we all feel like that in the beginning. It was during this placement that I first found my feet. Within the month I was feeling more able to assess patients undergoing surgery, taking them down to theatres and distracting them while they had their cannulas inserted and their anaesthetic administered; something that can be very daunting for a young person, let alone their parents and families. Caring for a child post-operatively was something I was feeling more confident at as the weeks went on, ensuring that they are able to eat, drink and mobilise alone before discharge, and recognising when things maybe weren't going to plan and alerting my mentor of any concerns I had and recommendations to improve the situation. I was also given the opportunity to watch surgical procedures in theatres, which of course I took. I was able to watch a tonsillectomy, a myringotomy and insertion of bilateral grommets.

Whilst being in that environment was nerve-wracking, with all the monitors beeping, surgical staff surrounding the patient, and some degree of blood, I felt helpless in the fact that, if I was needed to do something, I would not have known how to help, but the surgeons and anaesthetists were so understanding, explaining everything they were doing and encouraging me to come to conclusions about the rationale of their actions. As a student, this has remained so beneficial to me. I was so thoroughly supported by all staff on this placement, nursing and medical, and will always consider it as the best introduction to the world of nursing I could have possibly received.

Towards the end of my first year, I was given a four week placement in the Adults Outpatient Department at Essex County Hospital. Despite being a paediatric nursing student and initially being a little disheartened I'd been given an adult nursing placement, I had an incredible time with the staff nurses, health care assistants and doctors during my time there. I was able to work on my communication skills with a variety of patients, and gain more experience in dressing wounds using an aseptic/sterile technique. Despite this experience being on leg ulcers (something not ordinarily seen in children), this skill is transferable and I have since been confident dressing wounds on paediatric patients. In the dermatology clinics I was also able to assist in minor surgical procedures such as biopsies, removal of suspicious or unwanted skin lesions, and removal of stitches, something I really enjoyed. Looking back now, especially after this year's decision to transfer all services and close Essex County Hospital, I am so glad I was able to work in such a beautiful, historical building. The first year flew by quicker than expected, and this continued through my second and final years.

Second year began similar to the first. We spent the first few months in university again, having more lectures and skills sessions.

We were able to spend time together as a cohort and exchange experiences and knowledge.

My first placement in my second year I was placed in the Children's A&E department. I have always had an interest in the environment of A&E and emergency care, enjoying television programmes such as BBC's Holby City and Casualty and being a trained first responder within our Scout Group. You soon realise once you are actually in the real A&E environment that it isn't entirely like what you see on the TV. Again, on my first day, I was assigned a mentor and was orientated around the department, having a look through the resuscitation area and the adult minors and majors departments too. My first misunderstanding during this placement was what the staff in A&E expected of me. Being a second year student, I had an increased responsibility. I thought the staff working with me would expect me to know things and do things that I wasn't sure I knew myself. But in fact I found it to be the complete opposite, I was given a couple of weeks to find my feet, shadowing some incredible staff members and building my confidence. Soon, I was triaging patients and discussing with my mentor what I would diagnose. I was beginning to confidently administer medication such as oral pain relief, nebulisers and oxygen therapy.

On programmes and films about life in A&E you will frequently see the "red phone"; the emergency phone in the resuscitation area where paramedics alert the resus team of who they are bringing in and their expected arrival time. This time could be fifteen minutes, but it could also be less than five, giving the team little time to prepare the area for what could possibly be coming through those doors. As a student, I was able to observe and sometimes be involved in these emergency calls, be it trauma, cardiac or respiratory arrest, uncontrolled seizures, sepsis or meningitis. I can't deny I was petrified when the patient was bought in by the paramedic team, they gave the handover and all of a sudden it feels like there's 100 staff surrounding the patient, gaining various IV accesses, attaching leads upon leads and listening as alarms go off, all while speaking to the patient and telling them what they were doing and why. Sometimes as a student, all you can do is stand back and watch, and be the one to comfort the family. But as the

Ooh Matron!

weeks went on, I did feel more comfortable passing blood bottles and fluid bags to the doctors, documenting observations every five minutes and trying to get a history from the patient or their family.

I feel I learnt a lot from my time in A&E, increasing my knowledge of acute care and emergency situations. I also experienced placements in the community with the paediatric outreach team, an insight into children and adolescent mental health, and spent some time with the school nurses and health visitors, all whilst completing assigned essays and a graded presentation in front of my class and tutors. Second year, much like the first, flew by.

Which brings me to my third year, the final year! Now that nursing training is a degree, (whereas before you could complete it as a diploma), students are required to write a 10,000 word dissertation based on an element of research within their field. Throughout the first two years, this word 'dissertation' is thrown about, and all students begin to ask themselves if they are capable, a thought that crossed my mind several times throughout my training. I won't lie and say it was easy. Writing a dissertation while juggling 30 hour weeks on placement, days at Uni, and at least trying to have a social life and hold down a part time job, is hard. Despite placements becoming a little 'easier' in the third year, because at least you almost know what you are doing and can begin to work under your own initiative, I would still class the third year as the most difficult. On top of the dissertation, we also had three exams, one scenario based, one multiple choice and one medication calculation; all of which require a lot of time for revision and preparation. So while the stresses of placement are reduced slightly as you begin to feel more comfortable in practice, the stress of the theory work is overwhelming. A lot of the time as a student, I thought to myself, "Surely I will learn everything I need to on placement, so why the need for all this theory work, exams and lectures?" The knowledge and skills obtained throughout the three years of training are theory bound. That's the foundation of what we do, we wouldn't be able to practice as nurses without knowing the reasons why we do things; the reasons behind monitoring blood pressures in renal patients, the reason behind why a suppository is inserted one way and not the other, the reason behind inserting an intraosseous cannula as opposed to a peripherally inserted venous cannula.

I'm at the end of my third and final year, currently on placement on the Children's Ward, where I will be starting as a Staff Nurse after my training. I've completed almost 2300 hours of practice on placement and a similar amount in University. Do I feel like a nurse? Yes, I'm now having my own patients to look after on shift, administering their medications, monitoring their input and output and organising their plans of care. I'm handing over my patients to the next team who will be caring for them. Even though I'm at the end of my training, I'm not in any way at the end of my learning. There's still so much I need to learn and will experience as a qualified nurse, and I am thoroughly looking forward to the next part of the journey.

A nursing degree is not like any other degree. I may be biased saying that, being a nursing student, but I truly believe it. The breaks from university and placement are short. Depending on where you study you get 4 weeks in summer, 2 at Christmas and 2 at Easter. The working days are long and unpaid, the assignments and study hard. You'll finish a 12 hour shift, go home and get straight back to studying, finishing your essay or finding more research articles for your literature review, when all you want to do is rest. But you won't find a single nurse; adult, paediatric or mental health, who will tell you it's not worth it. Three years is a short time when you consider what you learn. But the learning doesn't stop there. Nurses will continue to learn throughout their lifelong career, new research will come out and policies and procedures will change. You'll meet people, patients and their families who will teach you and inspire you. Your outlook on life will change, and you'll find yourself smiling at the end of your shift. Not because you get to return home and finally empty your bladder, take your shoes off and enjoy a cup of tea, but because, as clichéd as it sounds, you know you've made a difference to someone, somewhere. I've loved my time as a student nurse, through the good days and the bad days. I'm lucky I've had someone like Sarah to turn to when I needed advice or just someone to talk to if I ever needed it. She's shared her knowledge and experiences with me through the last

Ooh Matron!

three years and I couldn't thank her more. She may feel she hasn't helped, but just knowing someone is there is always enough, and I am very much so looking forward to being able to continue sharing my experiences with her as a qualified paediatric nurse.

Sarah Jane Butfield

Chapter thirteen:
Accident and Emergency beckons

Now for something completely different. Who puts their hand into the food processor to push the food down instead of using the plunger? Well, I think we have all probably done this to some degree, however one woman did it in style with the blades turning. Her husband, shocked by her screams and the blood stained appliance he saw when he went to her rescue, became a patient himself. One look at the food and blood mixture in the food processor bowl caused him to faint and so his wife had to call an ambulance to collect them both. He hadn't lost consciousness, but he was vomiting. On admission we were unsure whether it was due to his concussion or the sight of his wife's bleeding hand as the ambulance crew applied a temporary dressing in the ambulance after removing the tea towel she had applied at home. She very proudly announced on arrival in the A&E department that while waiting for the ambulance she had picked the pieces of skin from the food mixture, which was supposed to have been done in case we might want or be able to sew the pieces back on! They looked like flakes of cooked white and red cabbage.

Of course we could not attempt reattach any of them and fortunately for her the damage to her hand was superficial and limited to her skin and two fingernails, although it would be very painful for some time afterwards. Her husband made an embarrassed but full recovery. As they waited for their discharge letters before getting a taxi home his wife delighted in making sure everyone in the waiting area knew he had fainted!

The younger staff in the department, me included, were less experienced in dealing with the guaranteed procession of Saturday night drink related accidents and incidents that would come through the door. This one speciality, due to the timing of it in our training, meant we were permitted to do two weeks of night duties, so there would be no escaping the increased police presence, angry intoxicated patients and their visitors. Security staff operate in the

Ooh Matron!

A&E department at a much higher resource level these days than they did in the mid-1980s and so I learned from the best. The senior nurses on night duty included three large rotund ladies who worked permanent nights. They operated a zero tolerance of bad language or intimidating behaviour in the department. Drunk men seemed to think that a buxom older woman would be maternal, ready to take care and mop their brow. NO. Sew them up and ship them out was the order of the night especially on Fridays and Saturdays. The wives and partners of drunken men nearly always protested too much about the perceived 'insensitive treatment 'of their loved ones, even though very little of the experience would be recalled the next day. The more serious drink related incidents often resulted in police hanging around to take statements or to escort people to the police station for questioning when they were given the all clear for medical discharge. This police presence also often inflamed the tension in the waiting areas.

The things they can't teach you about emergency nursing can be hard to deal with. For me, the time in A&E meant dealing with my first cot death, also called Sudden Infant Death Syndrome (SIDS.) Unlike today we rarely, unless it was a major incident, had any information about what would be arriving by ambulance in the A&E department. On arrival the patients were immediately triaged and directed to either the emergency area often referred to as 'resus' for acutely ill, life threatening injuries, etc., or to cubicles for those requiring assessment, initial treatment and review. The waiting area housed the walking wounded who would be called to be seen as and when a treatment room or cubicle became available. Cot deaths and acutely ill babies or children always went straight through to resus. The most disconcerting image for me when the eight month old baby girl arrived was that she looked like she was sleeping, but had been attacked with the insertion of intravenous drips, cannulas and attached to monitors, while completely unperturbed by the interventions. The enormity of what had occurred and what remained unresolved was demonstrated the moment the mother walked in. Drained of all colour, crying, but with eyes wide searching for hope and on the verge of hysteria, she was unable to control the insidious shaking that overwhelmed her. The father, trying to remain strong and in control, tried to comfort the mother with little success, tears breaking through as he turned his head towards the resus area.

I had never expected to be allowed to enter the resuscitation area during such an extremely sensitive and traumatic medical emergency but my mentor insisted that this invaluable learning opportunity in both nursing and pastoral care should not be missed and so I followed her in. With no children of my own, my only experience had been when I worked with babies on the children's ward and obviously newborn babies at the maternity hospital, which bore no comparison to this situation. I stood well back so that I could see and hear everything happening from a medical standpoint. However, I also felt compelled to observe the mother, who had been allowed in. I was in awe of the way the staff cared for her as if she were an individual patient and not the mother of a baby undergoing resuscitation. The history revealed that the baby had been found floppy and unresponsive at home. The baby had been given CPR (Cardio Pulmonary Resuscitation) at the scene, initially by the parents and then by the ambulance crew. Despite this, on arrival at A&E, the medical and paediatric team worked on the baby for a further thirty minutes before finally 'calling it' and stopping the CPR. As if synchronised, the mother was led away with a firm arm around her shoulder moments before the resuscitation stopped. She collapsed within a few steps, quickly being scooped up by the staff who were escorting her and placed onto a trolley bed. Totally overcome by the emotion, sadness and distress of the parents as it played out in front of me, I found myself crying. I immediately felt guilty for intruding on their grief. However, as I looked around I saw that many other members of staff had tears falling down their faces or watery eyes waiting to burst. Within minutes the baby, devoid of monitors, drips and oxygen masks, was wrapped in a white hospital blanket and handed to its mother, just as they do in the labour suite after delivery, this scene so far removed from the happiness of that first embrace. The father, now lying beside the mother, placed his arm around mother and baby as they cried and stroked her as if she still had life in her small body.

Over the years SIDS and its possible causes, contributory factors, behaviours or social prevalence has been widely researched and reported on. When high profile celebrities such as Anne Diamond, who lost her son to SIDS in 1991, became involved, awareness improved and her contribution to the 'Back to Sleep' campaign saw her work recognised by the Royal College of Paediatrics and Child Health. Cot death is still one of the major concerns to all parents, new or experienced. Now, as a new grandmother, I am acutely aware of it when my grandson stays over at our house.

There were relatively few surgical procedures that a student nurse was deemed competent enough to undertake independently. However that all changed when I lost my trephination cherry! After initial training in this procedure was complete, the trephination of nails was one which commonly presented in A&E and therefore gave a third year student nurse like myself plenty of practice. As much as I longed for the opportunity to work autonomously the act of nail trephination was not exactly what I had in mind.

The definition of nail trephination is the surgical procedure used to release the pressure in the nail bed by drilling a hole (trephining) through the nail into the hematoma. Trephining is generally performed using a heated needle which is passed through the nail into the blood clot.

The medical term for a blood clot under the nail or a bleed into the nail bed is 'subungual haematoma'. Nail bed injuries can be caused by trauma to the finger or toe nails. Drainage of the blood from the nail bed, by trephination, relieves the pressure and the acute pain associated with it.

The first one that I completed solo, completely unsupervised, was on a builder whose right thumb had been injured by a masonry hammer. He presented with a purple black discoloured nail and there was evidence of the nail slightly lifting from the nail bed. He had been examined by the triage nurse, had his thumb x-rayed to exclude any fractures and as there were no lacerations to his thumb the protocol at the time was to try and preserve the nail by trephining.

As I set up my dressing trolley with the dressing packs, saline, povidone iodine antiseptic skin solution and most importantly the needle, my nerves began to kick in. In the innocence of youth I still assumed that all builders, especially large burly tattooed ones, were as 'hard as nails,' as they say in Suffolk and that they could take any pain inflicted on them. I had seen Keith's builder friends break bones at Sunday morning football matches and still try and continue playing. Therefore I felt reassured that my patient would not cause me any problems unlike a recent female patient who had a nail trephined by one of the triage nurses and screamed louder than a woman in labour!

The man was in a cubicle on a trolley bed behind a set of curtains. Carefully opening the curtain with my elbows, after washing my hands, I set about placing the blue surgical drape over his arm and chest so that I had an aseptic working area. As he was a large man and the trolley height was not adjustable, being just under 5 foot 5 inches I was overstretching in every move I made. The setting up went well and he chatted and made small talk although I had to ask him not to laugh as his belly movement almost dislodged my drape. As I replaced my gloves and picked up the sterilised needle and turned towards him he rolled off the opposite side of the trolley. Quickly getting to his feet and struggling with the curtains, he tried to make his escape. He didn't say a word. I put the needle back on the trolley and followed him out into the waiting area and then into the car park where he stopped, out of breath and said, "Bloody hell girl, what did you think you were going to do with that bloody great needle?" He paused and took a deep breath and I wondered if he was going to faint. "You said you were sorting out my nail, not giving me an injection!"

The misunderstanding suddenly became obvious. After a great deal of reassurance and further explanation of the procedure, including the use of the needle, I did eventually trephine his nail. Contrary to his expectations he didn't feel any pain just a slight pressure on his nail. He was very apologetic before leaving the A&E department and he returned an hour later with a big bunch of flowers for me and a tin of Quality Street chocolates for the nursing staff to share.

Chapter fourteen:
The Anatomy of becoming a qualified nurse

On one of my trips home to Ipswich in 1986 as I was preparing for my final examinations I was talking to my friend Sandra who I had known since secondary school. She had married and started a family while I completed three years training. I found myself talking about the struggle to find enough time to revise and how having such a wide variety of conditions, disease, scenarios, etc., to cover felt quite overwhelming, when she suddenly said, "Ha, all these years I thought you'd taken the easy option going off to train as a nurse. You nurses always make it look like it comes naturally and is more about common sense."

Those words jumbled around in my head. Did she genuinely have no concept of what the role of a student nurse might involve and what a student nurse might need to learn? I thought, maybe saying it out loud does make it sound rather unbelievable, especially when you reel off the list of wards and places you've worked such as: accident and emergency, medical, surgical, obstetrics and gynaecology, psychiatric, orthopaedics, paediatrics, operating theatres, community nursing and the list goes on. Could it be that people outside of nursing and health care might have perceived me and my role as just a fun-loving student nurse? In hindsight it is easy to see why it might have looked easy, however it was far from easy. Yes we had fun and I made some amazing friends, but I also worked hard on my studies whilst in the ward environment experiencing happy, sad and eye opening experiences. The reality was and still is that the view from the outside is rarely the same as the view from within.

In my three year training period an air of change started to develop and it focused on student nurses and their training providers. The way training was delivered, together with the way students' knowledge and skills were assessed and examined, was part of an ongoing review and the early signs of a new more academically led training regime were evident.

Our class became some of the first student nurses to take a combined multiple choice and essay length final examination and, looking back over my transcript of training, it's difficult to conceive now how we managed to fit so much into three years. My training commenced on 10th October 1983, with my general State Final Examinations being held in November 1986. The final results and registration came through in December 1986. For just over three years my life as a student nurse led me into a variety of wards, specialities and community based settings, with the sole aim of providing a rounded insight into nursing and a baseline of nursing and medical education. At the time I did not realise that this was just the beginning. The misconception is that you complete three years of training and become a nurse and your career is spent using that knowledge. The truth is far removed from this. From the day you qualify as a nurse the real learning begins and the reality is it that it never ends until you stop practicing. New procedures, medicines, diseases, policy changes, etc., are all part and parcel of ongoing professional and career development. And contrary to popular belief, it's not just ambitious go-getters who have to keep learning, it is every nurse, in every setting, because nothing stays the same. The needs of patients, their medical conditions and treatments change continuously and as a profession, nursing must change, accommodate and keep up to provide high quality evidence based nursing care.

What does it take academically and practically to qualify as a nurse?

The nuts and bolts of my training and evaluation consisted of four practical assessments spread over the three year period followed by the Hospital and general State Final Examinations.

These practical assessments were categorized as follows:

- Aseptic technique,
- Administration of drugs,
- Total patient care,
- Communication & organisation known as ward management.

I totally under-estimated, when I started my training, how much preparation, practice and tension would be attached to these practical evaluations. I think it was because my perception of other students who had completed some or all of them was that it's just the ward sister watching you complete the tasks and giving you the thumbs up, and a pass, of course. However, for me the experience was nerve-racking and intense, or maybe I was just unlucky with the ward sisters I had for some of my assessments.

For the aseptic technique, you choose a patient with a wound that needs a dressing performed and then you complete this aseptic dressing procedure with the ward sister observing. Sounds simple enough. I had no issue with completing aseptic technique dressings, I was more worried about the other part to the assessment which was the knowledge check. This meant having to know the patient, their medical history, the background to the wound you intended to treat and apply a dressing to and their medication and ongoing care. I had picked a female patient who had a cholecystectomy or gall bladder removal. The way the consultants always referred to the patients at highest risk of needing this procedure was as 'fair, fat and forty'. As a young woman I found that funny, it's obviously not so funny when you reach your forties if the looks fit! The ward sister drilled me on my patient for thirty minutes although it felt like a lot longer; it felt as if the only thing she didn't ask me was the patient's shoe size.

With the experience and tension of the first assessment clearly implanted in my subconscious, my apprehension for the administration of drugs assessment was even higher. This was a much more in-depth assessment. I would be completing the ward medication round with my second nurse checker, adhering strictly to the hospital policies and procedures for safe administration of medicines. The ward sister would be observing and I had to know the action and side effects of every medication I dispensed. As students we were often the checkers on the medication rounds, therefore the additional preparation for this assessment meant going through all the medication charts of our patients in the days prior to this and ensuring that we knew every medication that was prescribed and in our trolley, but that's not all. I also needed to know about procedures for storage and administration of Controlled Drugs such as morphine and pethidine, what to do if there were missing medications, and how to proceed if an administration error was made, for example, wrong patient or wrong drugs given. On the day of the assessment, although I had prepared as much as humanly possible, I was not prepared for a change of ward sister or the number of new admissions overnight, whose medication charts I would have no time to look at thoroughly before my assessment began. Wouldn't you know it? Only five patients into the assessment, I meet a new patient with medication on their chart which I had never heard of. I pulled out the well-used ward copy of the BNF (British National Formulary) from under the trolley and began to look it up. At this point the ward sister walked away and I wasn't sure how to proceed. So I found the drug in the BNF and on my notepad made a note of the name, dose and contraindications then looked at the medication chart again. Happy that I knew what the medication was for and that the prescribed dose was within normal parameters, I closed the lid, locked the trolley and walked over to the ward sister who was at the nurses' station. Before I had a chance to say anything she said, "I'll be back in a moment, but you obviously know what you're doing so this will not take long." The sense of relief was overwhelming and with my confidence lifted the remainder of the medication round was uneventful. In the ward sister's office afterwards as the final questioning began I suddenly realised that I could do this. I had retained the knowledge and had been able to recall the facts required to operate safely as a nurse. I think this was the moment when I started to believe that I would finish my training and I would qualify as a nurse.

The assessment I enjoyed the most, if you are supposed to enjoy an assessment, was my total patient care. It is extremely rewarding to select a patient with a condition that not only interests you, but that will give a sense of satisfaction because the care that you plan has a positive effect on the patient's physical, psychological and emotional wellbeing. Although I wanted to complete this assessment on one of my general surgical ward placements where patients regularly were admitted with acute conditions, treated surgically and went on to make a full recovery which made a

Ooh Matron!

rewarding care package, my assessment was destined to take place on the female geriatric ward, described in earlier in this book. Even though it did not have the positive, happy ending I hoped for, it gave me an excellent way to describe the holistic care required in a longer stay setting which consequently incorporated many elements that I would not have considered in the acute ward setting. For example the role and influence of the allied healthcare team including occupational therapists, physiotherapists and social workers.

My communication & organisation ward management assessment took place on the oncology ward. In my third year of training as a student nurse, and now a wife, this new dynamic to my personal life changed the way I approached my study, revision and my practical work placements. I had started to take some driving lessons, although to be honest I had no need of a driving licence. If I needed to go anywhere that my mum couldn't take me, Keith had always been there to take me. I soon realised that the timing of this new learning experience was ill thought through, as I did not have the time or the mental capacity to learn anything other than nursing, and so the lessons go were put on hold.

Ward 8, Essex County Hospital - Oncology Care and Treatment. That may have been the professional name for the unit, but the patients all referred to it as the cancer ward. The use of the word cancer, especially in relation to some types and locations of cancers, evoked fear and made emotions run high. On the ward, the senior staff encouraged us to use terms like oncology, tumours, lesions and treatment, but never the word 'cure'.

The ward cared for a variety of patients, spanning both sexes and ages from sixteen upwards. There was also a range of reasons and rationale for their attending or becoming in-patients. Radiotherapy, chemotherapy, surgical removal of tumours and lesions and much more meant that the staff needed a specialised knowledge and skill set on a practical level; but on a psychological level they also needed an ability to empathise without patronising. The fears of patients were never to be belittled. Fears of changes to body image, of surgery, hair loss, etc., carried a multitude of emotional issues depending on the sex and age of the patient.

From day one on this new placement the staff started to help me prepare for my management assessment or, as it is formally known, my 'communication and organisation practical' element. Known and referred to informally as 'ward management skills' this included the management of staff, stores and supplies, staff allocation, drug monitoring and ensuring high standards of quality, patient- focused, care delivery.

I completed my management assessment on 30th September 1986 on the early shift. Despite my intensive preparation over the previous six weeks for any possible eventuality that could occur that day, I didn't sleep well the night before. I arrived at work an hour early with pockets full of copious, hopefully helpful, notes. The shift would start with hand over from the night staff, followed by me, the nurse in charge, allocating the patients to the staff on the early shift. Luckily, with no one absent or off sick that day, I had one less issue to deal with. The consultant led ward round would start at 8.30 am prompt before the radiotherapy and planned surgical procedures of the day got underway.

As a general oncology ward we had a wide mix of patients suffering from various forms and locations of cancer. Some in-patients required respite care and not treatment, to give their family or carers some time off, although most families and carers still visited daily and participated in their relatives care. Other patients had been admitted for courses of chemotherapy which nowadays would be probably be carried out as day case treatments, but at that time required a hospital admission.

End of life care can be a very difficult concept to come to terms with and some of the patients with the more aggressive or advanced cancers had Do Not Resuscitate (DNR) stickers and entries in the hospital notes. These decisions, made on a purely individual basis and never taken lightly, were always completed after due consideration and consultation not only with the medical professional team and patient, but also the next of kin. It is essential in the ward and community setting that everyone involved is aware of the patient's wishes. Seeing a DNR sticker on the notes always gave me an uneasy feeling. We are trained to do everything possible to preserve life, so what would I do or how would I handle it if I saw someone developing Cheyne–Stokes respirations?

Ooh Matron!

Cheyne-Stokes This is when a patient develops an abnormal pattern of breathing characterized by progressively deeper and sometimes faster breathing, followed by a gradual decrease that results in a temporary stop in breathing, called an apnoea.

The knowledge that the development of this type of respiration pattern can often indicate the final breaths that the patient would take, sometimes lasting hours sometimes only minutes, was unnerving. We were not going to jump in with medication or artificial breathing aids, but instead we would ensure that the patient was pain free and keep them as comfortable as possible. The last hours of life are often spent with a loved one in attendance and therefore our role revolved around supporting them while giving them the space and time they need together.

During my management assessment, we had three patients with DNR orders in place, but fortunately all were stable and comfortable. The ward sister who conducted the assessment followed and watched my every move, making notes and randomly questioning me as to the rationale of various decisions I made throughout the day. As I write this now having had the experience of taking a driving test, I can compare my management assessment to the stress and apprehension of taking your driving test over six hours instead of one. All I dreaded was an 'emergency stop' which would mean I had made an error of judgement that needed a senior member of staff to intervene and take over. The consultant ward round had gone smoothly, and the registrar was very kind in making his writing more legible for me in the patients notes and on the medication charts afterwards. This helped me to avoid any errors or mistakes that might have impacted on my performance. The staff all worked hard and efficiently, and I am sure in hindsight that they saved me on a couple of occasions from schoolboy errors due to nervousness as they put words in my mouth about possible action to take to resolve issues on the ward. Strangely on this shift, we didn't run out of anything, no one came back late from their coffee or lunch breaks and no staff bickering could be heard anywhere. A huge sense of relief came over me when the ward sister said, "Come to my office so that we can review your performance." I knew the end of the assessment was in sight, I was on the home stretch. Would I cope when I had to manage a ward full of staff and patients alone? And would I always be lucky enough to have such support from the medical, nursing and ancillary team behind me? The honest answer to the second question is, no. But that's a whole other story.

I passed my assessment with excellent feedback and the promise that, if a staff nurse position became available in the oncology unit in the future, sister would welcome my application. With my last practical assessment completed, the time had come for the final preparation for the hospital and state examinations. The reality of finally becoming a staff nurse moved a step closer, and it felt amazing.

The relief at passing my final practical assessment prior to focusing on my Hospital and general State Final Examinations was immense. Many wonderful people helped to get me through my final year, especially my fellow classmates Lorna and Teresa. Together we enjoyed copious amounts of coffee and chocolate biscuits during our revision sessions which did nothing for my waistline but the boost to my mental health at this stressful time was well worth the uncomfortable sensation every time I wore my uniform belt.

As I progressed through my training I thought that the four practical assessments that formed part of the nurse training syllabus were stressful enough, but I hadn't bargained on the intensity of the practical ward based competency assessments. These included practical skills that would be essential in my future role as staff nurse and eventually a mentor to future student nurses, even though as a student I could not ever imagine that I would or could put another student nurse through the pressure and ordeals created whilst gaining these essential skills. We had not only to learn the theory and rationale, but to gain the practical ability to perform these sometimes invasive and critical skills, which if not carried out correctly carried increased risks of complications including infection, damage to organs and structures, i.e. blood vessels, skin, etc., or worse still the death of a patient. They included:

- Naso-gastric tube insertion, care and feeding
- Male and female urinary catheterisation

- Care and management of suprapubic catheters
- Stoma care and evaluation, i.e. colostomy, ileostomy and urostomy
- Intravenous fluid management and cannula care
- Wound drainage management
- Blood transfusions
- Cardiac monitoring
- CVP lines (Central Venous Pressure) and the list went on.

Before I was permitted to carry out any of these independently or with only minimal checking and supervision required, there were periods of intense observation, questioning and then constant supervised practice until I was assessed and signed off as ready to manage patients and their skilled care needs independently. Mastering practical skills, although initially daunting, did become easier, as my mentors said it would, with practice. A bit like starting to learn to drive in that when you start driving lessons it takes a little while to settle into each lesson. You have to adjust the mirrors and seat, etc., drive around to rebuild the confidence since your last lesson then just as you are getting the hang of it the lesson is over. When the next one comes you start off hesitant again. If more than a few days passed between opportunities to practice my new skills that was exactly how I felt. However, as time went by my nervousness turned into self-belief, which in turn increased my self-confidence, and so by my third year of training the process of ward based learning had worked and I felt like a skilled practitioner. It was however at this stage, with my confidence riding high, that I met a challenge which was less testing of my skills with technical equipment and procedures but which challenged my powers of observation, assessment, and understanding.

A patient was admitted from home for a pressure sore assessment and possible surgical intervention. The district nurse team had discovered the pressure sore, which had been described to them as 'a bit of a sore bottom'. Why would something that sounded quite minor possibly need surgical intervention? The patient was female age about sixty years old and she suffered from Parkinson's disease for which she was taking the medication

Madopar. One of the characteristics of this disease is a slow, shuffling gait (walking) insomnia and memory issues. This patient, who we will call Jill, lived with her daughter who cared for Jill as she needed full-time supervision and care to maintain her safety. The district nurse team did not visit Jill as the patient on this occasion, but her daughter who had recently had a minor surgical procedure on her foot. As she was a large woman she couldn't reach her foot to redress the wound and so the district nurse was booked to do the dressing and check on the wound's progress. This was the second visit by the district nurse to attend to the wound and while she was there she heard crying coming from the bedroom. Upon questioning the patient, it was discovered that she cared for Jill and that 'she was having one of her turns' was the way the daughter described the reason for her mother crying. The district nurse asked to see Jill and when she went into the bedroom she was shocked to find her restrained in a child's single bed. When her daughter was questioned about this she said that she couldn't chase around after Jill while her foot was sore and so being in bed was the safest place. The district nurse went over to Jill and asked her what was wrong and her response was incoherent. The daughter said Jill had a bit of sore bottom and that she had been putting cream on it. The district nurse offered to take a look and when she unwrapped Jill and exposed her bottom she discovered an open pressure sore on Jill's sacral area which was oozing green slough mixed with blood. Jill felt hot to the touch and her skin was pinch dry and wrinkled. An ambulance was called and that was how Jill ended up in hospital.

After being triaged in Accident and Emergency she had been referred to the surgical team and arrived on the surgical ward. I was asked to admit her and assess her pressure sore before the surgical team visited her to make their assessment. It was difficult to complete the admission paperwork as Jill wasn't able to answer many of the questions and so I awaited the arrival of her daughter who had decided to come to the hospital with a neighbour instead of in the ambulance with her mother. As yet she still hadn't arrived. With the help of a first year student nurse we positioned Jill in the bed on her left hand side supported by pillows so that her bottom was relieved of any pressure and was visible for a thorough assessment. In the meantime, a baseline assessment was carried out.

Ooh Matron!

It is perhaps best if I describe the results more or less as they would have been presented.

Observations: Jill had a raised temperature of around 38 °C which indicated a possible infection. Her blood pressure was slightly low at 90/60 mm hg (millimetres of mercury) and her pulse was rapid and irregular at over 120 beats per minute.

An intravenous cannula had been inserted into her left arm in the ambulance and she had a one litre bag of normal saline in progress to combat dehydration and also to allow access for the initial intravenous antibiotics which had been prescribed and the first dose administered in the Accident and Emergency department. A baseline set of blood tests had also been taken to check for anaemia, electrolyte levels and white cell count, etc., and we were awaiting the results.

Nursing examination of the wound: Jill had an open wound on her sacrum which measured just over 3cms in width, undeterminable depth at that point. The purulent green slough, congealed in places, was swabbed for M, C & S (microscopy, culture & sensitivity) to establish if infection was present and which antibiotics it might be responsive to. After irrigation with normal saline via a syringe the wound bed could be properly examined. There were dark areas of necrotic, dead, tissue and only small areas of pink granulating tissue.

From this initial baseline examination it was apparent that this pressure sore had developed over a period of time and due to inadequate treatment it had subsequently become contaminated by the use of a barrier cream, far too late in the pressure sore's development and treatment, meaning it was now infected. I cleaned and covered the pressure sore with a loose dry dressing while we waited for the surgical wound review. By the time the surgeon and his entourage of junior doctors and medical students arrived to carry out the review, Jill's daughter had still not arrived. Therefore, with a limited medical history to work on, a non-invasive plan would be implemented. This involved me telephoning and following up by fax to request confirmation of Jill's medication and medical history from her family doctor so that we could cross reference it with her existing hospital notes. The broad spectrum intravenous antibiotic therapy which had been started would continue for a further 24 hours then convert to oral administration, subject to review when the wound swab results were available. If the results indicated antibiotic sensitivity to a different form of treatment then the regime type and route of administration would be reviewed and amended as/if required. As the decision in the initial assessment was not to resort to a surgical debridement of the necrotic tissue this meant we would implement a wound care regime of daily chemical debridement, irrigation and dressings. Jill would be in hospital for some time and therefore ongoing assessment commenced to ensure the correct levels of care and treatment were given.

In relation to Jill's pressure area risk, the assessment of choice in the 1980s, which we had been trained to implement and utilise, was the Norton scale originally devised in the 1960s. There were five areas of consideration. The patient's:

- Physical ability
- Activity potential
- Mobility
- Continence
- Mental awareness

Each area of consideration was given a rating between 1 and 4 and when added together if the score was 18 or more the patient was low risk. A score of 14 to 17 was a medium risk, 10 to 13 high and less than 10 very high risk. Several factors resulted in Jill being assessed as a high risk. First, since admission Jill had been incontinent of urine, although we did not know if this was normal for her or if it was stress and hospital environment induced. She had an existing pressure sore, was only just over 9 stone in weight (under 60kgs) and unsteady on her feet. On admission her mental awareness was impaired possibly by the admission to hospital, separation from her daughter and disruption in her medication regime.

With the clinical components of Jill's care and treatment now in place the big question was, 'where is her daughter?' Hours had passed since she was due to arrive with her neighbour and as there was no answer on the telephone number that we had for their home, the initial concern was that something had happened to her. As my shift drew to a close and still with no news, the ward sister decided that if they had not made contact with her daughter by the morning we would request that the district nurse visit to check on her. Jill, her condition and the story behind her admission played on my mind that night and I felt relieved to be heading back to work the next morning for an update. A message had been left with the district nurse team for someone to visit the house and to call the surgical ward with their findings so that we could update Jill, who by now was feeling better, tucking into her breakfast and had queried her daughter's whereabouts. A few hours later a call was received saying that the district nurse had found Jill's daughter and that she had requested that Jill not return home after her treatment, but be moved to residential home as she couldn't and didn't want to care for her mother any longer. This was a big shock to us all. The social work team had to become involved not only to visit Jill's daughter but over the coming days to make Jill aware of the changes that may lay ahead for her care. In hindsight, I now know it was my lack of life experience and incomprehension of a daughter behaving that way towards her mother that made it almost impossible for me to understand or to empathise. However, as I was told by my mentor at the time, and as I now know from personal experience, the world of a family member as a carer, if not properly supported and monitored, is fraught with danger. Many families struggle on, too proud or embarrassed to ask for help or to seek advice or guidance on how to care for elderly relatives with sometimes mentally and physically demanding conditions. Jill remained on the surgical ward for ten days and because her wound continued to respond well to the antibiotic and wound care regime, she was transferred to the geriatric ward for ongoing care and an eventual move to a residential home in Clacton. I found out later that during this time Jill's daughter started visiting her mother, a positive step for their future relationship.

Sarah Jane Butfield

Chapter fifteen:
Enter Staff Nurse Parker

Ongoing end of year written assessments, case studies, and the practical skill tests, at the tutor's discretion, culminated in the Hospital Final and the general State Final Examinations which took place in November. The formal presentation of our hospital badges and certificates took place in May 1987.

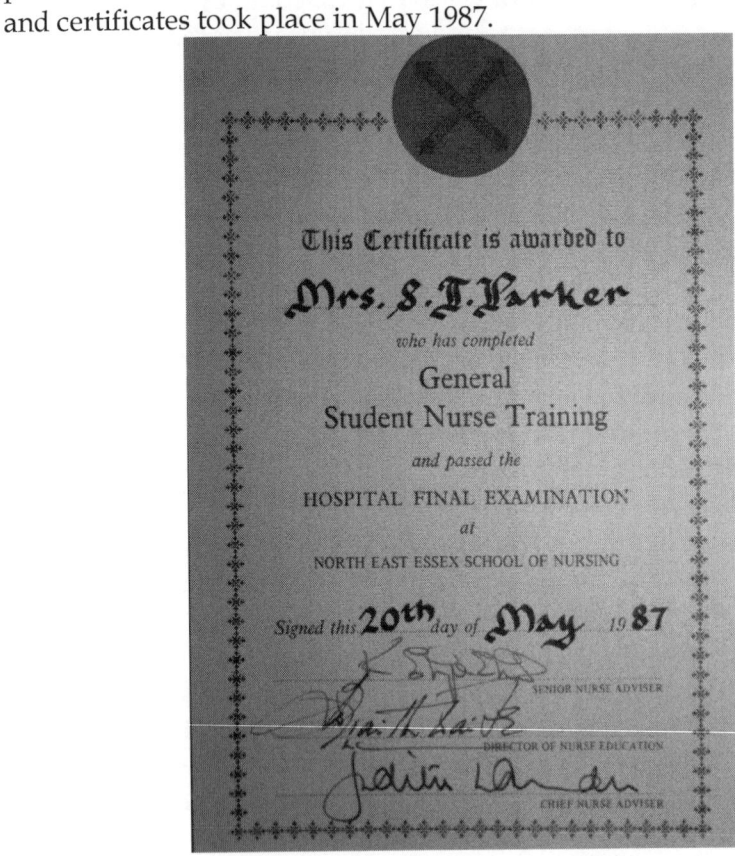

Hospital Finals Certificate

Between October 1983 and November 1986 I completed 2180 hours of classroom theory and 3325 hours of practical ward based placements, excluding overtime! With the completion of three years

Ooh Matron!

training, practical placements, assessments and passing the final written examinations it was time to register as a Nurse.

On 22nd December 1986, I received the long awaited results envelope. It contained two A4 size letters. One confirming that I had been successful in passing the State Final Examination which I sat on 24th November 1986. The second letter was my registration document which came with instructions to take it to the bank and pay the fee of £65 to commence the registration process. The final months of my training had been hard work with little time for any light relief. Even when the exams and assessments were over I did not dare stop studying in case I had failed and needed to re-sit any or all of the components. So to finally receive the official notification that I could now practice as a nurse after registering with the UK Central Council or UKCC as it was generally referred to, was an immense relief.

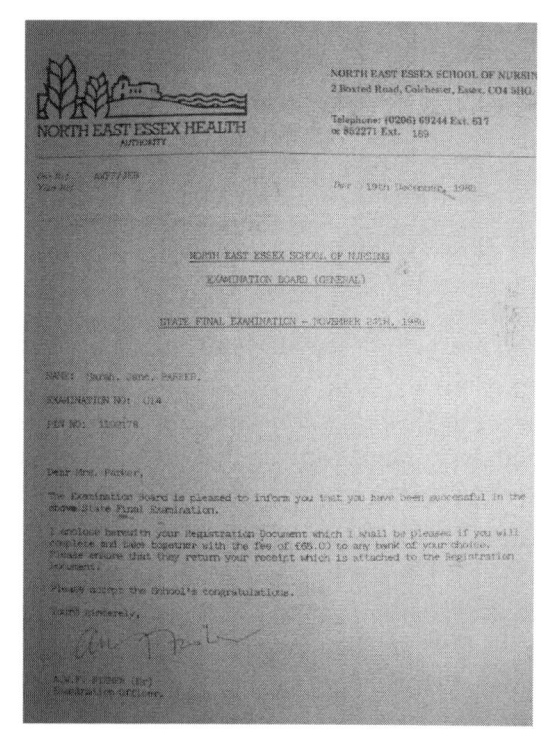

State Final Examination results confirmation

Sarah Jane Butfield

In the waiting time between taking the Hospital Final Examination and the State Final Examination we were encouraged to start applying for qualified nurse positions as junior staff nurses. Some of my friends had already decided to continue on with post graduate courses like midwifery and mental health, so they had no need to involve themselves in this process. However, those of us wanting to go straight into the workplace had to find a position in an area that interested us and go through the recruitment process. Before getting married in 1985, if anyone had asked what I wanted to do after qualifying the answer would have been simple, I wanted to train to be a midwife, but things had changed and so my plans for the next stage of my career changed too. I applied for junior vacancies on the surgical and gynaecological wards as I had enjoyed those placements, but because of the low number of vacancies versus the high number of applicants, my tutor encouraged me to apply to the geriatrics speciality which always had a high turnover of staff. I wasn't successful in obtaining a position in my preferred specialities, but I did receive the offer of a junior staff nurse position at St Mary's Hospital on the male geriatric ward. After the initial disappointment, I discussed it with my tutor, who reassured me that geriatric nursing was a great way to hone my management skills and that if I added six months post graduate experience to my CV then applying to other wards and units would be easier and more successful. Therefore I focused on these positive elements and moved forward.

Apart from when I got married this was the first time I had needed to deal with any kind of formal registration. The registration of nurses started in 1922 and after the 1943 Nurses Act, registration became compulsory. This is still a legal requirement for any nurses of speciality who wish to practice in the UK today, although since 2001, the statutory body of nursing has been the Nursing and Midwifery Council (NMC).

When I qualified in 1986 the UKCC worked alongside the four national boards, whose roles included overseeing the standards of education for nurses. It operated from 1983 to 2001. Prior to 1983, since 1921, three General Nursing Councils (GNC) covered the United Kingdom. They had documented duties and clear responsibilities for the training, examination and registration of nurses. GNCs also took responsibility for approving nurse training schools like Colchester School of Nursing and for maintaining the nurse register in each of the constituent countries. My national board was the ENB (English National Board). 1986, a time for change for nurse education, meant all new student nurses from that time would be part of the Project 2000 style of nurse education. This, one of the many reforms of the regulatory system for nurses, started and it sent ripples through the nursing profession over the next five years.

English National Board confirmation

With my registration paperwork completed and the fee paid my wait for my PIN number to arrive began. My excitement and relief, combined with the sense of achievement on completing my training was now replaced by a frustrating waiting period. I just wanted to work as a nurse, I had qualified after all. My personal insecurity lurked in the form of self-doubt. Would I remember all that I had learned if I wasn't practicing? During this period of waiting for my registration to be processed, I accepted the opportunity to start work as an auxiliary nurse on the male geriatric ward at St Mary's

Hospital where I would soon be working as a junior staff nurse. I would not be undertaking any nurse duties, although some of the nurses did take me as the second checker on the drug rounds that took place four times a day. These combined activities turned out to be a great introduction to the ward and the staff without the pressure of my new role. With the work of an auxiliary nurse easily within my skill-set, after three years as a student nurse, I remember being unprepared for the initiation and insight into the political agenda that existed in this grade of staff. The perceived 'them and us' divide, often hypocritical when face to face, between the qualified nurses and unqualified staff, which included the auxiliaries, porters and ancillary staff, was difficult to accept. I felt a bit intimidated by it to begin with because they all knew who I was and the reason for my working there in this temporary role. I was the newly qualified nurse who needed to make a good impression on all grades of staff, without compromising the responsibility and requirements of my role as I moved forward as a qualified nurse in few weeks' time. I was unsure of how they would treat or accept me. Would I be ignored and given the silent treatment or given a chance to be different? What actually happened was that they conspired to use this time to 'educate' me on how to treat and respect auxiliary nurses, tongue in cheek of course, but with the message strongly reinforced. I wondered if there were long-standing problems on this ward or in the hospital as a whole as I hadn't encountered this before during my placements or at least I didn't think that I had.

I became familiar with the layout of the hospital, the ward routine, some of the staff and their idiosyncrasies which would help me in the future. I had worked at St Mary's Hospital once during my training, on an eight weeks placement during my first year on the female geriatric ward.

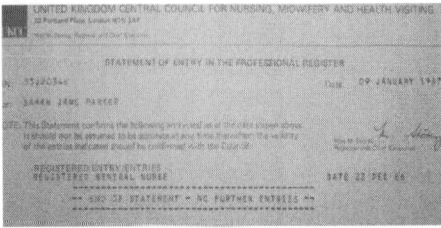

My Statement of Entry

Just after Christmas my PIN (Personal Identification Number) arrived and I began work as a Registered General Nurse. My excitement and eagerness to wear my qualified nurse navy blue belt adorned with my solid silver buckle, which I received as graduation gift, erased my nerves as the day approached for my first shift as a staff nurse. I worked my first shift as a qualified nurse on the 14th January 1987.

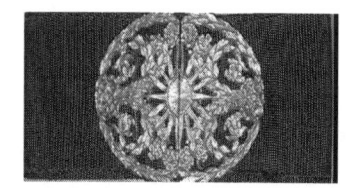

My silver nurse buckle

I was especially grateful for the short period as an auxiliary nurse when I saw the rota and realised that I had only three day shifts as a qualified nurse before going onto a set of seven night duties when I would be in charge of the ward! This was not how I expected it to be, so in that time I tried to gain as much information as possible about the night duty routines and what to do in an emergency, etc. The ward sister reassured me that she had every faith in my abilities and that the night sister would be keeping a close eye on me.

It was mid-January and the first of my night duties in charge had gone really well, I had two great auxiliary nurses to work with and the night sister who was a good resource. Jo the night porter popped in regularly to check on us and the 12 hour shift appeared to fly by. I arrived with confidence on the second night and all went well until we did the midnight 'back round.' This in house term meant going around with our trolley of linen, towels, incontinence pads, etc., and turning all of the patients who were unable to turn themselves. We would toilet them if necessary or change their incontinence pads and/or bedding if they were wet or soiled. Half way through the back-round we pulled the curtains around an elderly man's bed. He had been in hospital for a few weeks after suffering a stroke. As soon as I touched his hand I knew he was dead. Barbara, the auxiliary, put the over bed light on and we rolled him onto his back. He had cyanoses; blue, around his nose and mouth, but I checked for breathing anyway. No pulse, no chest movement and no breathing, definitely dead, Barbara fetched me the stethoscope to double check for heart beat but I heard nothing. We kept the curtains around him and although this was not my first death, I was shaking. I paged the night sister to come to the ward and we continued with the back-round. On arrival she checked the man and told me to call the duty doctor to come and confirm the death.

With the death confirmed by the doctor, at that time the protocol for performing last offices meant that the body would now be left for one hour as a mark of respect. Last offices is the term given to the preparation of the body before it is taken to the mortuary and then to the undertakers.

The procedure then included these basic requirements, although I have since come across many variations in this procedure. First of all we washed the body and administered mouth care and reinserted his dentures. As a male patient who was normally clean shaven, we shaved him as well. His eyelids were gently closed and we laid him on his back with his arms placed close in to him on each side. He had a couple of pressure sores and a skin break so we covered those with adhesive dressings. Fortunately, he didn't have any IV sites or any drainage tube entry points but if he had we would have covered these with gauze pads. All orifices are blocked if there is bodily fluid leaking. We attached a second hospital identification bracelet on the ankle to match the existing one on the wrist. If the mouth remained open we would sometimes place a rolled up clean white towel under the lower jaw for support. Finally we would dress the body, usually in a shroud, which we then wrapped in a clean white sheet around the body using a specific system of folds that ensured it remained tight and intact. An identification tag would be pinned to the sheet. This may sound macabre but in the geriatric setting I actually enjoyed performing last offices on our patients because they became like family and to be able to attend to them with such care one last time gave me personally some closure.

The next job was to check the notes to find out if the next of kin or family wanted to be contacted during the night or the following morning. As I flicked through the notes, with the night sister watching me, I was praying that they didn't want to be contacted as I really didn't know if I could keep my composure to deliver such sad news in a professional manner whilst still shaking and being quite overwhelmed by the event. My prayers were answered, he had been severely affected by the stroke, which was not his first, and his elderly wife and daughter had decided that there would be no purpose in them finding out during the night. I heaved a deep sigh of relief, and Barbara made a pot of tea for us to drink while we made our plan for the next stage in the proceedings. It needed a plan because performing last office required two staff so we needed to make sure no one was on their break and that the night sister was free to be on the ward in case another pair of hands were required or medication was needed by another patient.

When the last offices were completed the night sister paged Joe the porter to come and collect the body. Now, to properly picture the scenes that are about to unfold, you need to firstly remember that it's January, a cold and icy night. Secondly St Mary's Hospital is built on Balkerne Hill therefore the grounds to the back of the hospital slope downward quite steeply in places. Thirdly, the dead man is now dressed up from head to toe in a crisp white bed sheet looking like an Egyptian mummy with a pink carnation from his bedside flower arrangement taped to his chest. Added to which as we lift him into the tin trolley that is used to move the body to the mortuary we discover he is too long. Lastly the mortuary is situated at the back of the hospital down the hill, in outbuildings not attached to the hospital, so there is no way to access the mortuary internally.

We were all standing looking at each other having laid the man's body precariously half in and half hanging over the trolley.

"You can't go like that," said the night sister, "you can't even put the lid on!"

"It's ok." said Joe, "I will unscrew the bottom plate, then his feet can go through and I will put it back together afterwards."

We waited while he went to the porter's office to get a screwdriver and I got my coat as I had to accompany the body to the mortuary. Eventually the body was in the trolley and we were ready to go. The night sister took charge of the ward until my return.

As we made our way through the corridors to the side exit door Joe was at the head end and I was walking along at the side. At the exit into the drive which lead to the mortuary Joe said, "You might want to hold onto the trolley. I don't want you sliding down this hill."

There was not a lot to hold onto but I secured my grip on the side rim where the lid goes on and we continued. It was treacherous underfoot and even though I had my trusty, nurse shoes with plenty of tread on, I could feel myself sliding. Joe struggled to keep the trolley in a straight line and almost lost his footing as we hit something, not sure what it was. Anyway as he recovered his footing, still holding the trolley it tilted downwards, like he had released a lever or something. Suddenly the body was leaving the trolley through the foot hole! In that split-second I let go of the trolley to make a grab for the body and slid over, although luckily I was able to grab the sheet which stopped the body falling out completely. It was now part in the trolley with the legs end resting in my arms against my chest as I sat on the ground. At this point I was crying, not because I might be hurt from the fall but because of the horror of what had happened. Whenever I have told this story people are usually laughing so much at this stage that they fail to appreciate my feelings at that time, however I must admit that while writing about it I am sitting here smiling, ok sometimes laughing to myself, but it was not funny at the time.

"Shit" said Joe, "Are you alright?"

"Don't worry about me, get this poor man back in the trolley."

"Ok, but we will struggle to do this alone on this ice. I need to go get some help will you be ok there?"

"Well I'm not going anywhere unless we start to slide again, am I."

Ooh Matron!

Joe left, although not very quickly as he had to carefully navigate his way up the slippery hill to get some help. Soon I could see him returning with two people I didn't know, I couldn't see their uniforms because of their coats, so I was none the wiser of the positions they held at the hospital. Suddenly laughter broke out. They thought this was funny. I was so angry.

"For Christ sake get over here and help me", I shouted, feeling shocked at their disrespect of the position the dead body was in.

"Ok luv we got this", said one helper, who I could now see and hear was a man.

The three of them lifted the body back into the trolley and once he was safely inside they positioned themselves so one that one of them was holding his legs, Joe was pushing and after picking me up the other one held the side of the trolley with one hand and me with the other as we continued our journey to the mortuary. All I could think about now was telling the night sister and the fact that I would probably lose my job just as quickly as I had started it.

I needn't have worried about telling the night sister because by the time we got back to the ward everyone was talking about it, apparently an auxiliary on another ward had been having a smoke break and saw the whole thing and spread the word so the others could look out of windows and fire doors at the spectacle unfolding outside.

Back on the ward the night sister took me into the office and checked my wounds, well bruises and scrapes, saying very little. I think she wanted to give me chance to calm down. I discovered afterwards that apparently this was not the first time this had happened, although it was the first time on ice with a nurse ending up on the ground. The trolley was replaced immediately and to my knowledge it never happened again. I am pretty sure that Joe took the brunt of the blame and some form of disciplinary action because nothing was required of me other than to complete an accident form for my injuries. I was given four nights off and when I returned nothing more was said about it. So there we have it the culmination of three years training is celebrated in style with an incident within my first week as a staff nurse. Was this the way my nursing career was going to continue? I hoped not.

Sarah Jane Butfield

As I moved onto the next stages in my nursing career, which has spanned twenty eight years, I have accrued many more stories, anecdotes and experiences that I would like to share with you. If you have enjoyed this first book in 'The Nomadic Nurse series' I look forward to welcoming you back in book two, which has a working title of 'Bedpans to Boardrooms'. I move into my qualified nurse role and find myself working in aged care within the private sector whilst juggling my nursing career, pregnancy, motherhood and being a good wife.

Don't miss a book two excerpt after the extras at the end of this book.

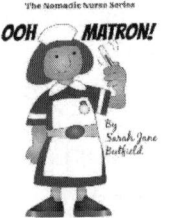

Thank you for reading the first story in The Nomadic Nurse series. Reviews are hugely important to authors and to future readers, so if you enjoyed 'Ooh Matron' and would like to leave me a review on the site where you purchased your copy that would be greatly appreciated.

Sarah Jane

Ooh Matron!

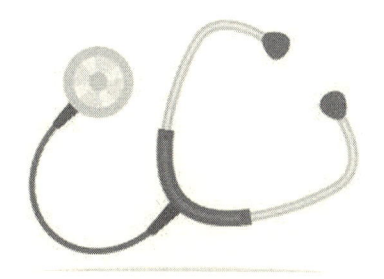

Medical Terms
Glossary

Do you love nursing or medical memoirs, but get frustrated by the acronyms and medical language that halts or interrupts your reading?

I have tried to include information in the narrative of the book to prevent that from happening, but as a backup I have added this medical glossary reference tool. If this has been helpful, or not, your feedback would be appreciated for future books in this series because as my career develops so does the technology, specialities and medical language. Feel free to email me at sjbutfield@gmail.com with your comments.

Catheterisation: An aseptic procedure where a thin flexible tube is inserted into the patient's bladder to drain urine.

Cholecystectomy: Surgical operation to remove the gall bladder.
Coeliac Disease: A disease of the small intestine causing hypersensitivity to gluten which in turn hinders food digestion.

Colostomy: The surgical formation of an opening from the colon onto the surface of the body, which functions as an anus.

Congenital Heart Defects: the term used for birth defects which inhibits the functionality of the heart.

Cushing syndrome: A metabolic disorder whereby the adrenal cortex over produces corticosteroid hormones resulting in high cortisol levels which causes weight gain, thin skin, muscle and bone weakness.

CVA: Cerebrovascular Accident or stroke – lack of blood flow to the brain caused by blood clots or haemorrhaging (bleeding) which can result in damage and possible death of brain cells. Signs and symptoms can include paralysis, speech impairment and cognitive changes.

Cystic Fibrosis: an inherited faulty gene disease that affects the movement of fluid and salt in the cells of the body resulting in the clogging up of lungs and the digestive tract with mucus.

Debridement: the removal of dead infected or damaged tissue.

D&C: Dilation and curettage.

EN: Enrolled Nurse qualification achieved after two years practical and academic training.

ERPOC: Evacuation of Retained Products of Conception.

Grommets: A grommet is a small tube that is inserted into the eardrum to allow air to enter the middle ear.

Gynaecology (Gynae): medical and surgical care dealing with the functions and diseases specific to the female reproductive system.

Hydatidiform: Mole: the development of a mass in the uterus made up of tiny fluid-filled sacs, hence the Latin name hydatid meaning drops of water, around an aborting embryo.

Hyperemesis Gravidarum: nausea and sickness associated with pregnancy.

Hysterectomy: Surgical operation to remove the uterus/womb.
Ileostomy: An ileostomy is where the small intestine is diverted through an opening in the abdomen.

Intraosseous cannula: A needle inserted into the bone marrow which provides an access route for the administration of blood, fluids and medication or for taking laboratory specimens when intravenous access is unavailable or contraindicated.

Intravenous: Within or into a vein.

Ooh Matron!

Lupus: An inflammatory disease affecting both the skin and internal organs.

Madopar: Medication used to reduce, control and treat the symptoms of Parkinson's disease by increasing the dopamine levels in the brain.

Microscopy, Culture & Sensitivity: The laboratory test carried out on specimens to detect, identify and try to establish a sensitivity to treatment.

Myringotomy: A small incision made into the eardrum to relive pressure caused by an excessive accumulation of pus or fluid in the middle ear.

Naso-gastric feeding: A naso-gastric tube is passed through the nose and nasopharynx into the oesophagus ending up in the stomach, to allow liquid feeds to be administered.

Nebulisers: A piece of equipment that turns a liquid, such as Ventolin medication for asthma, into a mist to be inhaled by the patient.

NHS: National Health Service created by Aneurin Bevan on July 5 1948.

Obstetrics (Obs): The area of medicine that deals with pregnancy, labour, and the puerperium or post-natal period.

ODA: Operating Department Assistant no formal qualification required in 1980's now replaced by qualified Operating Department Practitioner's.

Oophorectomy: Surgical removal of one or both ovaries.

Periodontal: Dental term for the tissues and structures around the teeth. Disease in this area can affect teeth, gums, jaw ligaments and bones.

Phrenology: is the study of the skull to determine a person's mental capability and character.

Postural hypotension: A form of low blood pressure that can occur when moving from a sitting or lying position to standing up.

Pre-eclampsia: A condition sometimes developed during pregnancy causing high blood pressure, proteinuria, headaches and fluid retention.

Psychiatry: Deals with the diagnosis and treatment of mental health disorders.

Pupil Nurse: Training to be EN.

RGN: Registered General Nurse – this replaced the title SRN.
Sacral area: The area covering the sacrum which is the bone at the base of the spine.

Sepsis: An infection in the body caused by pus-forming bacteria.
(SIDS) Sudden Infant Death Syndrome: also known as Cot Death is the sudden, unexpected death of an apparently well baby.

Sleep apnoea: A sleeping disorder characterised by periods when sufferers stop breathing for more than 10 seconds at a time.

Suprapubic catheter: Is a flexible tube inserted via the abdomen below the navel that is used to drain urine from the bladder.

SRN: State Registered Nurse qualification achieved after three years practical and academic training.

Student Nurse: Training to be SRN/RGN

Tonsillectomy: Removal of the tonsils which are located in the pharynx. (Back of the throat).

Triaging: A process whereby patients are clinically assessed into groups based on their medical needs and urgency for treatment.
Urostomy: A surgically created stoma or artificial opening for the flow of urine from the body.

Ooh Matron!

Step back in time
From the home of psychiatric experiments to student nurse education centre

A student nurse's view of the history of Severalls Hospital, Colchester

As a young girl brought up surrounded by farms, fields and small villages in Suffolk, the only time that I can remember being made aware of or noticing buildings was on school trips or when attending the local churches and chapels for Sunday School meetings or later with the Girl Guides. I think that studying the History of Nursing as a pre nursing student in Ipswich first stimulated my interest in the variety of nursing and healthcare establishments, especially those of the Victorian and Edwardian eras. Since then my curiosity has revolved around buildings of the past and the present and how the provision of nursing care was inextricably linked to the design of the buildings themselves. For example, there was the Nightingale ward layout, named after Florence Nightingale, which I witnessed and worked in at a variety of hospital locations. Many older hospitals, not specifically mental or psychiatric ones, had been designed around this ward plan that allowed for easy unobtrusive observation of all patients from a central point, unlike today's modern hospitals with smaller bays of six to eight beds, and single and double rooms. It wasn't until I moved to Colchester, and with a slightly more mature outlook in relation to my local environment that I began to realise and absorb the new found beauty in the buildings I studied and worked in and their significance to my new career pathway.

In Colchester, my interest in the history of the hospitals themselves developed from not just wanting to know and understand how the wards and nurses would have operated, but how the hospital as a whole derived its functionality from its design. Colchester has a long and colourful history in healthcare and hospital provision for both general and psychiatric care. In chapter six I gave you a brief insight into the history and background to the development of Myland Hospital in relation to its origins as an isolation hospital, built in the Severalls Hospital estate which encompassed an area of 300 acres. The estate was sold to Essex County Council in 1904, however the origins of Severalls Hospital itself date back to when construction started in 1910 and its subsequent official opening in May 1913.

When I first arrived at Severalls Hospital in October 1983 to collect my accommodation key, the first thoughts were in relation to the sheer size of it. It appeared to be sprawling, in a highly-organised almost regimented fashion, within its own perimeter walls. I am not referring solely to the hospital, and its associated buildings, but the size and expanse of the grounds. Little did I know or comprehend at that time what three hundred acres looked like or how many buildings and services it could accommodate. This was in direct comparison to the relatively smaller sites of the Ipswich Hospital and units where I completed the majority of my pre-nursing placements. Although Severalls Hospital was not a secure site, in terms of the grounds at that time, as a newcomer it was difficult to work out how far the open lawn areas and footpaths extended. Each day I would walk across or around the huge lawn and tree-studded grass areas, adjacent to Mill Road, on my way to an early shift or when attending the school of nursing buildings within the complex, and there was rarely anyone to be seen as the majority of hospital traffic entered from the main road entrance in Boxted Road. The style and design was unlike any hospital I had worked in before with the possible exception of St Clements Hospital in Ipswich, which I had visited during my college years. This was one of the Suffolk asylums of the late 1800s however it was much smaller accommodating only two hundred patients when it was operational.

The original Severalls Hospital, designed by Frank Whitmore & W.H.Town, was based on the 'Echelon Plan.' This style of hospital/asylum layout became popular throughout the UK during this period for its practicality. This design meant that the hospital was built around a network of long corridors, which from an aerial view resembled an arrowhead. However, on a practical level it made all the essential services accessible without exiting the building therefore increasing security yet giving the asylum an open feel, an important element in mental health care even back then. Severalls Hospital varied slightly from the mainstream Echelon plan in that by the 1920s-30s it began to incorporate colony style, standalone villas in the grounds which accommodated staff, special services and later the academic services. The villas were built in the Queen Anne style, with few distinguishing features. However, there was a clear distinction in the extra styling and adornments, denoting the importance of the occupant to be. This was most apparent in the construction of Larch House and Severalls House probably because the latter would have been the Medical Superintendent's home.

Severalls Hospital oozed intrigue, but with a curious charm that endeavoured to hide its dark history. Psychiatric hospitals of the late 1800s, and early 1900s were steeped in horror stories of false imprisonment, ill-treatment and notoriously poor living and working conditions for staff and patients alike. It's quite sad in retrospect that some of the perceptions of psychiatric illness and care which originate from those times have left their mark on the way mental health issues in the elderly are perceived and dealt with in today's society. I think it is easy to forget sometimes that many of today's 70 to 90-year-olds will have first-hand knowledge and memories of family or friends affected by the institutionalised care and conditions of the asylum days.

The other feature meant that, unlike today, patients were separated not according to their psychological, medical or surgical needs but by their gender. What also made this hospital estate even more individual was that, apart from the design which kept all the wards and services linked, it was also self-sufficient in many respects as it had its own electric power producing equipment and two farms which operated within the three hundred acre estate to supply all the food required by the patients and staff. They bred their own livestock, grew their own vegetables and crops and even had their own in-house bakery.

The remit for Severalls Hospital was for it to become the second Essex County Asylum. The first Essex County Asylum was situated in Brentwood, and was known as the Warley Asylum. This name

Sarah Jane Butfield

remained until 1920 when it became the Brentwood Mental Hospital. The specification for this second asylum was that it should be able to house up to 2,000 in-patients at any one time. It was destined to be more than merely a group of psychiatric wards because with the Echelon design it formed a complete community of buildings and services for staff and patients. No one would ever need to leave. Many patients lived the remainder of their lives in the hospital and very few left except in a coffin. Institutions for 'mental defectives' were also labelled, 'Asylums for idiots, imbeciles and the feeble minded', which gives an indication of how people inadvertently became patients. It was not unusual for female patients to be placed in these institutions by their families as a result of pregnancy out of wedlock, being victims of rape or suffering from what we now know as post-natal depression.

One of the major architectural features of the estate was its chimney which was apparently lowered in height during World War Two reduce the risk of interfering with aircraft damaged in warfare trying to land at the nearby RAF Birch and RAF Boxted airfields. However, if you ask anyone who has ever worked or visited Severalls Hospital to name one thing that sticks in their mind, the chances are they will mention the corridors. This is not purely because they were a major feature of the design, but from an internal perspective in days gone by and during my time at the hospital, they were imposing, haunting and incredible architectural features. Over the years many people have documented stories about the hospital, its staff and patients and many of these articles and books make mention of the original corridors having no windows just openings which exposed the people using and working in the corridors to the weather. When windows were added the corridors still featured highly as stories told of staff using bicycles to travel between wards and departments due to the time it took to walk them and of bats flying freely and staff running and screaming to escape them. For me it was the noises that echoed through the corridors when no one appeared to be around that triggered not only my imagination, but also my apprehension. Many ghost stories exist about the hospital, its past inhabitants and their treatment. Most of these stem from the well documented use of

Ooh Matron!

these patients in psychiatric surgical and medical experimentation during the 1950s.

It is not uncommon to read and discover that, in mental hospitals and institutions throughout the UK during the 1950s, psychiatrists performed experimental treatments and procedures on their patients, practices which would be considered barbaric in modern times. These procedures included early forms of electro-convulsive therapy and even frontal lobotomies without sedation or anaesthesia. The introduction of phrenology around that time, and the belief that the shape of a person's head could indicate mental defects, encouraged the curiosity about brain functionality and the brain make up of these perceived social deviants.

After the NHS was established in 1948, county hospitals worked in groups to supply essential services for their local residents. Severalls Hospital, also part of this new organisational structure of hospital provision, saw the introduction of a small section of general services within the Severalls estate, including a new operating theatre, a medical ward and later two further general wards. In the 1960s, a period of change started that affected the management of psychiatric hospitals and the training of nursing and medical staff and ultimately this led to a more humane approach to treatments and therapies. The introduction of visual and auditory therapies such as art classes and movement to music sessions complimented the more appropriate prescribing, monitoring and regulated medicating of patients and their rehabilitation programmes.

As the protocols for long-term care for people with mental health care conditions continued to change over the years, the need for large institutions diminished as their care packages moved towards the community. For this reason many hospitals that started out as asylums ultimately were ear marked for closure. Although still operating as a combined psychiatric and general hospital during my student nurse years at Severalls (1983-1986,) by the 1990s, only one section remained open to inpatients and that was a ward to treat and rehabilitate stroke patients and the elderly. In March 1997 Severalls finally closed its wards and doors with the final patients being transferred to Colchester General Hospital.

Sarah Jane Butfield

If you are interested in viewing other people's images of the derelict Severalls Hospital site here are a couple of good articles.

http://www.slate.com/blogs/atlas_obscura/2014/05/30/severalls_hospital_is_an_abandoned_mental_institution_in_essex_england.html

http://www.ukurbex.com/index.php?/topic/946-severalls-asylum-mile-end-colchester-jan-2011/

Sarah Jane Butfield

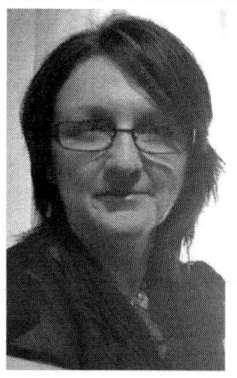

About the author

Author Sarah Jane Butfield was born in Ipswich, and raised in rural Suffolk, UK. Sarah Jane is a wife, mother, ex-qualified nurse and now an internationally published author. Married three times with four children, three stepchildren and two playful Australian Cattle dogs, she is an experienced modern day mum to her 'Brady Bunch', but she loves every minute of their convoluted lives.

Sarah Jane, the roving Florence Nightingale, fulfilled her childhood dream of becoming a nurse and went on to use her nursing and later teaching qualifications to take her around the world. She is now an international best-selling author of three travel memoirs set in Australia and France. In addition, she released Book 1, The Accidental Author, from her new 'What, Why, Where, When, Who & How of Book Promotion Series' for aspiring and debut self-published authors in February 2015 with Book 2, The Amateur Authorpreneur released in May 2015.

Sarah Jane loves to connect with her readers so feel free to connect on Facebook, Twitter or on her author website.
http://sarahjanebutfield.wix.com/sarahjanebutfield
Twitter @SarahJanewrites
www.facebook.com/AuthorSarahJaneButfield
www.facebook.com/Twodogsandasuitcase
www.facebook.com/OurFrugalSummerinCharente

Ooh Matron!

Travel Memoirs

by

Sarah Jane Butfield

Sarah Jane's travel memoirs are available at online bookstores worldwide, all links are available on her author website at http://sarahjanebutfield.wix.com/sarahjanebutfield

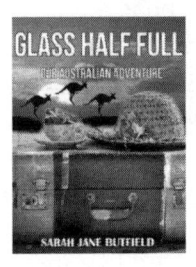

Glass Half Full: Our Australian Adventure

Is the glass half-empty or half full? Ironically, sometimes life influences our view and alters our perception.

When a UK step-family makes the tough decision to seek a new life in Australia it appears all their troubles are over as their new life begins. Life in Australia exceeds their expectations until challenging life events including grief, loss and relationship issues test their powers of positivity, persistence and determination. However, a bigger test was coming. When they lose their home, assets and belongings to the Brisbane floods in January 2011 they have to decide when enough is enough! A touching true story that many readers will relate to.

Sarah Jane Butfield

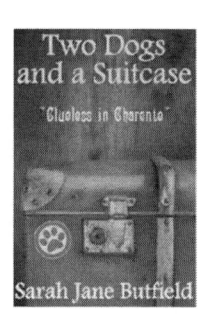

Two dogs and a suitcase: Clueless in Charente

The title says it all: what we have and where we are. This book, the sequel to Glass Half Full: Our Australian Adventure, follows our French exploits as we endeavour to rebuild our lives in another new country, after spending four and half years in Australia. Our goal, or hope for the immediate future, is to focus positively on the present, so that we can start a new, optimistic future back in Europe. Our main aim is to be nearer to the children, leaving the dark clouds of the challenges we faced in Australia as a distant memory. Journey with us as we arrive in rural South West France; enjoy my reflections, thoughts, and observations about my family, our new surroundings, and our lifestyle. Follow the journey of my writing career and how we start our renovation project while managing our convoluted family life. Once again, we will laugh, cry, and enjoy life to the fullest with a generous helping of positive spin thrown in for good measure.

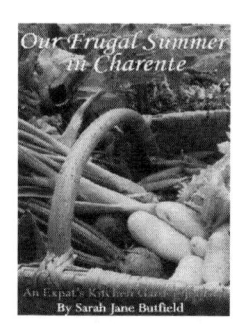

Our Frugal Summer in Charente
Voted one of the top 50 self-published books worth reading 2015`!

Ooh Matron!

Voted Self-Published Book Worth READING
www.ReadFree.ly

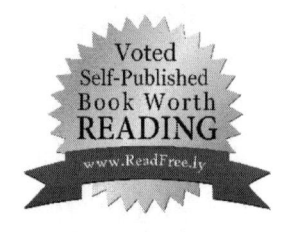

Meet Sarah Jane, a woman with a reputation for culinary catastrophe who tries to keep her family fed in challenging circumstances in rural France. Frugal living was not part of the plan when they arrived from Australia to undertake the renovation of a quaint cottage in the Charente. However, when life throws them a curve-ball the challenge was set. How to survive in France with very little money and two Australian cattle dogs. The answer came in the form of 5 chickens, 4 ducks and a vegetable garden! The frugal plan was to save money by any means possible, to enable any money they could earn to be invested into continuing the renovation of the cottage. In true 'Good Life' style Sarah Jane attacks this challenge head on by keeping some small livestock and converting a garden, that resembled a meadow, into a French 'potager' or kitchen garden. The French tradition of using produce from their 'potagers' is renowned for enabling families to create meals that are healthy, cost effective and simple. There are 31 recipes for a variety of food and drinks, included in a month by month account, of how they transformed a neglected garden into a frugal yet productive expat kitchen garden.

Photobooks to accompany the travel memoir series

Book 1 Views Through My Lens: Hobart and surrounding areas.
Permanently free at all bookstores

http://sarahjanebutfield.wix.com/sarahjanebutfield

Taking up photography, as a cathartic exercise, after losing almost everything to the Brisbane floods in 2011 gave Nigel a different perspective on life and his Australian surroundings. There

Sarah Jane Butfield

is an old saying that a person's eyes are the "window to their soul." We have found that our photographs are the window to our memories. This is the first book in a series from places we have lived, visited and enjoyed which we hope will appeal not only to followers of our adventures, but also to people who are interested in photography or travel.

Photobook 2 *due for release later this year.*

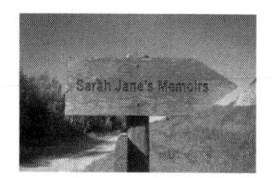

To have first access to subscriber only photographs and to hear about Sarah Jane's latest books, author events and great competitions, sign up for Sarah Jane's Memoirs -Author Sarah Jane Butfield's Personal Mailing list (no spam ever).
http://eepurl.com/0IuML

Chat with me and other memoir authors and readers at We Love Memoirs:
https://www.facebook.com/groups/welovememoirs/

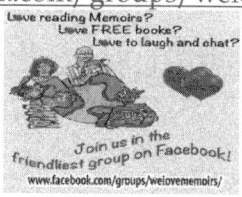

Other books by Sarah Jane Butfield

The Accidental Author

This is book 1 in a new series which looks at self-publishing for beginners and the skills needed for ongoing book marketing and promotion. This e-books series is based on the experiences of author Sarah Jane Butfield who writes travel memoirs, non-fiction books and romance short stories.

The Accidental Author introduces the author and this series of self-help e-books for new or aspiring self-published authors. The introduction starts with how and why Sarah Jane came to write and self-publish Glass Half Full: Our Australian Adventure. Find out how an aspiring author aims to be discovered while learning on the job how to write, publish and launch a new career in writing. Beta reader Shontae Brewster says, "A must read for any aspiring author or readers interested in the life of a self-published author. Sarah Jane's never give up approach to life and anything she turns her hand to is beyond admirable."

The Amateur Authorpreneur

The Amateur Authorpreneur is a beginners' guide for authors who intend to develop their writing into a business, addressing the important task of book promotion and marketing. We look at laying the foundations of the authorpreneur book promotion toolkit, building a fan base on social media and much more.

You've written a book or you plan to - what do you need to consider?

What does it offer readers?
Why will they buy it?
Where are your readers?
When will you publish it?
Who are you?

Sarah Jane Butfield

How do you promote it!
Find out how to take the business of being an author up a gear to become an authorpreneur.
The Amateur Authorpreneur will describe, using the What, Why Where, When, Who & How template, the process of taking the first steps into combining the craft of being an author with the business of marketing your work.
Here are some beta reader comments:

"Aspiring authors will feel reassured that whatever their age or IT ability all of the skills needed to become an authorpreneur are achievable."

A non-author beta reader said, "I have discovered skills and tips that now helps me in both my personal and professional social media interactions."

An avid reader who enjoys the work of indie authors was, "amazed at what's involved behind the scenes."

Available at all bookstores here
http://sarahjanebutfield.wix.com/sarahjanebutfield

Sneak preview
Bedpans to Boardrooms!
Excerpt from chapter one:
At the helm of my new career as an RGN!

I soon settled into the role of junior staff nurse at St Mary's Hospital. It gave me a new routine in both my work and home life, as a young married career woman. At the age of twenty-one with a husband of thirty-two it was not long after qualifying as a nurse that the question of having children arose. My new nursing career lay ahead of me now, but I also wanted a family. Of course, I had always been aware that at some stage the age difference would mean compromise by both of us. We would both want different things from our married life at different times. So finding some common ground would take negotiation. Whatever happened and whenever we decided to start a family, one thing was for sure, I had to complete my six months post registration period as an RGN. If not I would have no hope of working in the NHS acute sector on my return to work. What was I even thinking about? How would I return to work after having a baby? From a financial viewpoint, there was no doubt that I would have to return to work. We had just sold our one bedroomed starter home in Wivenhoe and moved into a two-bedroomed house on the same estate, as we loved it there. With no extended family living nearby to be able to help with childcare, if a return to work needed to happen changes at home and at work would be essential.

So how would I steer my career forwards knowing that I would need to interrupt it at some point to start a family? No idea. I still harboured aspirations of completing my midwifery post graduate course. However, the eighteen-month course plus examinations could not be interrupted for maternity leave. As I continued working I constantly reviewed my options. Even though the male geriatric ward was a great place to work and an ideal place to hone my skills as a junior staff nurse, I was ready for a new challenge.

Sarah Jane Butfield

In May 1987 two things happened to focus my attention on my home and work life balance. The first was that the ward sister on Ward 8, the oncology ward where I undertook my management assessment, contacted me. Before I left my oncology placement the ward sister had said that if I was interested in a junior staff nurse position, and one became available, she would invite me to apply. If that happened it would be a huge honour and a great opportunity for any first year staff nurse. Therefore, when the ward sister from Ward 8 called to let me know that such a position would shortly be advertised and she wondered if I would be interested my answer was, 'Hell yeah!' Well those weren't the exact words I used in that telephone conversation as you can imagine. I monitored the internal notice boards at every break time for the internal vacancy listing and the reference number needed for my application. At last it appeared and I was off, like the proverbial ferret up a drainpipe, to submit my application. This was achieved with the help of my mentor, the ward sister on the male geriatric ward. She recognised my ambitious streak and realised that I needed more than her ward could offer me. I knew that her ward was renowned for a high turnover of qualified staff, the main reason being that there was, at that time, no clear career pathway or progression. With my application submitted, the waiting began. Would I be shortlisted for an interview? I was pretty confident that I would, after all she did invite me to apply. In May I received a letter informing me that I had been successful in being selected to attend an interview on Ward 8.

The second thing that happened in May was that I was on sick leave from work with a stomach upset. I suspected it was due to the Chinese meal we ate the previous night after my late shift. I had been feeling nauseous all night so something I ate obviously didn't agree with me. Despite being unwell the news that I had an interview lifted my spirits. I spent the day re-reading my oncology notes on policies, procedures, treatment regimes, etc. I wanted to be well prepared and get the job I wanted. I would be off work for a further two days with this lingering stomach bug so I decided to take advantage of the sunny weather and read in the garden. Reading always made everything feel better.

Ooh Matron!

On my return to work I was still not feeling 100%. I was in the sister's office preparing the patients' notes for the doctor's ward round. With no explanation Babs, one of the auxiliary nurses, a large African woman, rushed in and hugged me. She held me so tight she almost restricted my breathing.

"Oh my lord, praise the lord!" She said as she released me. "Our little Sarah has the look of motherhood about her."

"What are you talking about Babs?"

"You're glowing beautiful girl. When are we gunna be hearing the patter of those tiny footsteps?"

"I'm not pregnant Babs, I had a stomach bug that's all."

"When was that? I didn't even know you were sick little one."

"Then why did you think I was pregnant?"

"I can see it in you. Here give me your hands?"

She took both my hands and held them tight with her eyes closed. "I see a beautiful baby girl." she said.

As she opened her eyes and released my hands I looked at her and for a split second I wondered if she was right. Could I be pregnant? I tried to dismiss the thought as Babs put her arm around my shoulder.

"Sorry if I've upset you Sarah. I inherited this talent from my mother, just as she did from her mother."

"I'm fine Babs honestly, I'm just a bit taken aback. Don't worry, when and if I get pregnant you will be the first to know."

Babs hugged me again and left to resume her linen trolley duties.

The rest of the day passed quickly with no more talk of babies. However, on the way to catch the bus home my conversation with Babs replayed over and over in my head. Unintentionally the next thing I did was to walk into the chemist and buy a pregnancy testing kit. I would do the test the next morning and then let Babs know that her baby radar was a bit off course on this occasion.

The presence of one blue line would indicate no pregnancy hormones in my urine. Two blue lines and I'm pregnant. As I sat in the bathroom holding the white plastic testing kit, which resembled a flattened white board marker pen, I realised that I did not have any method of timing the test. I had got out of bed, determined to use my first urine specimen of the day for the most accurate result, forgetting that my watch was on the bedside table. I didn't want to walk around holding the test, Keith did not know I would be taking a test as I didn't want him to get excited for no reason. I could hear myself counting: one Mississippi, two Mississippi, three Mississippi. We used to do that at school, playing hide and seek, that was until I realised how ridiculous I sounded. I looked down planning to find somewhere to place it while I went to get my watch but there staring back at me already were two thick blue lines. Oh my god Bab's was right, but would she be right about it being a girl? Well I would have to wait a while to answer that one.

I didn't know what to do. Should I tell Keith now or do I make an appointment to see the doctor to have it confirmed and then tell him? Yes, definitely that would be the best thing to do, tell no one until the visit to the doctors. With no doctor's appointments available to fit in around my shift pattern until a week's time, I decided to put the result of the test to the back of my mind as I now faced another dilemma. Should I still attend the interview on Ward 8?

I decided that I should still go to the interview by convincing myself that it's possible to get a false positive on a home pregnancy test. How gutted would I be if I wasn't pregnant and I passed up the opportunity of attending the interview? However, on the day of the interview pangs of guilt invaded my thoughts. I think being in denial up until this point about the pregnancy suddenly gave way to the deep down knowledge that I needed to accept it and face facts. I not only suffered from the morning, well actually all day, sickness and nausea, but I had this strange tingling sensation in both breasts. I also needed to pee almost hourly and on more than one occasion I wondered if I might have a urine infection instead of a positive pregnancy test. I couldn't pull out of the interview at this late stage or it would be obvious that I had known for a little while. So I psyched myself up and headed off to Essex County Hospital. The 45-minute interview with the sister from Ward 8, and another ward sister that I didn't recognise, went better than I could ever have imagined. I managed to answer their questions with relative ease. As the interview progressed and my confidence grew I focused so much on how well it was going and how much I wanted

Ooh Matron!

the job that all thoughts of a possible pregnancy completely disappeared.

I am still not quite sure how I managed to keep the news of my possible pregnancy from spilling out of my mouth as there had been so many opportunities to say something that week, both at home and at work. Babs kept randomly hugging me which thankfully none of the staff thought anything of, as she was a very tactile woman. Some close friends of ours announced that their first baby would be due in November, and with a guilty heart I concealed the possibility of our own baby news. Well at least for a short while longer until I was one hundred percent sure. At last the doctor's appointment. The treatment room nurse took my urine sample and did their equivalent of the home pregnancy test. The test involved test tubes like the ones we used on the gynae ward during my placement there during my second year of training. "Congratulations, you're pregnant," that's all I heard. The next thing I remember was being handed an appointment card for a blood test and a booklet about antenatal care. Despite having ample time to get used to the idea of being pregnant, I still walked home in a state of shock. However, by the time I reached home I was smiling with a sense of relief. Then the sensation of pure love for my unborn baby rushed through my body, mind and spirit. All thoughts of work and careers gave way to thought of prams, cots and an overwhelming desire to tell the world!

Keith, as expected, was over the moon when I told him the news, as were both of our families. At work I didn't know when to announce it, but for the health and safety of myself, my baby and my colleagues it needed to be soon. At that time we still manually lifted patients and frequently used 'The Australian Lift'. This was a two nurse manoeuvre that involved putting your shoulder under the patient's armpit while facing the top of the bed. Then clasping wrists under the patient's thighs with your partner before lifting them up the bed. This put a huge strain on your neck and back muscles. The crouched position would become increasingly uncomfortable as my pregnancy developed and there was no way I was going to risk losing my baby. So, at the earliest opportunity I told the ward sister who immediately relieved me of all lifting duties. Babs, the one person I wanted to share my news with, was on annual leave. I didn't like that everyone else on the ward was finding out about the baby before her as I had promised she would be the first to know. I need not have worried. Babs returned to work with a 'Congratulations' card and a beautiful pot plant called a cyclamen. With my pregnancy hormones in full flow my tears of happiness fell frequently.

A week later the letter, which previously I would have anxiously awaited, but now had completely forgotten about, arrived. It was informing me that my application had been successful for the position of junior staff nurse on Ward 8 at Essex County Hospital. Now the reality of deciding how I would manage my career and a family started to kick in. I would need to return to work, if only for financial reasons. We had a mortgage that could not be covered by one income especially with a family to support. These events all occurred during the 1980's property boom. I made a conscious decision that I would not let worrying about what might happen after my baby was born spoil my pregnancy. Therefore I took a very blinkered view of we will deal with that when and if the time comes, ever hopeful that things might change. After a period of sick leave for hypertension or raised blood pressure I started my maternity leave and Samantha Louise was born on 7th December 1987. She was born three weeks early in an induced labour after I developed pre-eclampsia, a complication of pregnancy which demonstrates itself with symptoms including hypertension, swelling (oedema) and protein (proteinuria) in my urine due to the extra strain on my kidneys.

Not long after the birth, I needed to consider how and when I would be able to make a financial contribution to our household income. The only skill that would earn me the maximum amount of money for the least amount of hours worked was nursing. All of my maternal instincts told me to stay at home with my new baby, but the need for me to return to work in the months that followed did not abate. Even so I would not contemplate working fulltime and so when I did return it was not to my job in the NHS. Instead I would now have my first experience of working for a non-profit organisation providing aged care services in nursing and residential homes in Colchester. I became a part time (weekend) staff nurse at

Ooh Matron!

Cheviot Nursing Home. A new development in my career waited in the wings, preparing to open up, although for me at the time it was just a new part time job to make ends meet. Little did I know what lay ahead.

To be continued!

Book 2 is due for release in 2016

Printed in Great Britain
by Amazon